Gastrointestinal Cancers and Personalized Medicine

Gastrointestinal Cancers and Personalized Medicine

Editors

Stefania Nobili
Enrico Mini

MDPI • Basel • Beijing • Wuhan • Barcelona • Belgrade • Manchester • Tokyo • Cluj • Tianjin

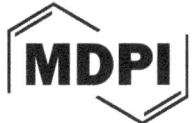

Editors
Stefania Nobili
Department of Neurosciences,
Imaging and Clinical Sciences
"G. d'Annunzio" University of
Chieti-Pescara
Chieti
Italy

Enrico Mini
Department of Health Sciences
University of Florence
Florence
Italy

Editorial Office
MDPI
St. Alban-Anlage 66
4052 Basel, Switzerland

This is a reprint of articles from the Special Issue published online in the open access journal *Journal of Personalized Medicine* (ISSN 2075-4426) (available at: www.mdpi.com/journal/jpm/special_issues/gastrointestinal_medicine).

For citation purposes, cite each article independently as indicated on the article page online and as indicated below:

LastName, A.A.; LastName, B.B.; LastName, C.C. Article Title. *Journal Name* **Year**, *Volume Number*, Page Range.

ISBN 978-3-0365-3808-2 (Hbk)
ISBN 978-3-0365-3807-5 (PDF)

© 2022 by the authors. Articles in this book are Open Access and distributed under the Creative Commons Attribution (CC BY) license, which allows users to download, copy and build upon published articles, as long as the author and publisher are properly credited, which ensures maximum dissemination and a wider impact of our publications.

The book as a whole is distributed by MDPI under the terms and conditions of the Creative Commons license CC BY-NC-ND.

Contents

About the Editors vii

Stefania Nobili and Enrico Mini
Special Issue: "Gastrointestinal Cancers and Personalized Medicine"
Reprinted from: *J. Pers. Med.* **2022**, *12*, 338, doi:10.3390/jpm12030338 1

Sonia Hermoso-Durán, Guillermo García-Rayado, Laura Ceballos-Laita, Carlos Sostres, Sonia Vega and Judith Millastre et al.
Thermal Liquid Biopsy (TLB) Focused on Benign and Premalignant Pancreatic Cyst Diagnosis
Reprinted from: *J. Pers. Med.* **2020**, *11*, 25, doi:10.3390/jpm11010025 7

Arianna Dal Buono, Federica Gaiani, Laura Poliani, Carmen Correale and Luigi Laghi
Defects in MMR Genes as a Seminal Example of Personalized Medicine: From Diagnosis to Therapy
Reprinted from: *J. Pers. Med.* **2021**, *11*, 1333, doi:10.3390/jpm11121333 27

Gaëlle Rhyner Agocs, Nazineh Assarzadegan, Richard Kirsch, Heather Dawson, José A. Galván and Alessandro Lugli et al.
LAG-3 Expression Predicts Outcome in Stage II Colon Cancer
Reprinted from: *J. Pers. Med.* **2021**, *11*, 749, doi:10.3390/jpm11080749 41

Noshad Peyravian, Stefania Nobili, Zahra Pezeshkian, Meysam Olfatifar, Afshin Moradi and Kaveh Baghaei et al.
Increased Expression of *VANGL1* is Predictive of Lymph Node Metastasis in Colorectal Cancer: Results from a 20-Gene Expression Signature
Reprinted from: *J. Pers. Med.* **2021**, *11*, 126, doi:10.3390/jpm11020126 53

Hossein Taghizadeh, Robert M. Mader, Leonhard Müllauer, Friedrich Erhart, Alexandra Kautzky-Willer and Gerald W. Prager
Precision Medicine for the Management of Therapy Refractory Colorectal Cancer
Reprinted from: *J. Pers. Med.* **2020**, *10*, 272, doi:10.3390/jpm10040272 75

Zsolt Zoltán Fülöp, Réka Linda Fülöp, Simona Gurzu, Tivadar Bara, József Tímár and Emőke Drágus et al.
Prognostic Impact of the Neutrophil-to-Lymphocyte and Lymphocyte-to-Monocyte Ratio, in Patients with Rectal Cancer: A Retrospective Study of 1052 Patients
Reprinted from: *J. Pers. Med.* **2020**, *10*, 173, doi:10.3390/jpm10040173 95

Roser Velasco, Montserrat Alemany, Macarena Villagrán and Andreas A. Argyriou
Predictive Biomarkers of Oxaliplatin-Induced Peripheral Neurotoxicity
Reprinted from: *J. Pers. Med.* **2021**, *11*, 669, doi:10.3390/jpm11070669 105

About the Editors

Stefania Nobili

Dr. Nobili is an Assistant Professor of Pharmacology at the Department of Neurosciences, Imaging and Clinical Sciences of the "G. d'Annunzio"University of Chieti-Pescara (Italy). She achieved her Pharm.D. degree at the University of Rome 'La Sapienza'in 1989, her Specialization in Applied Pharmacology at the University of Florence in 1997, and her Ph.D. in Chemotherapy at the University of Milan in 2001. In 2013, she was awarded the Alberico Benedicenti Award for Pharmacology and Toxicology from the Italian Society of Pharmacology. From 2007 to 2019, she worked as an Assistant Professor of Pharmacology at the University of Florence (Italy). Her research interests are focused on the preclinical and clinical pharmacology of anticancer drugs, in particular, cancer pharmacogenetics and pharmacogenomics and tumor drug resistance, with an emphasis on the drugs used in the treatment of gastrointestinal neoplasms.

Enrico Mini

Enrico Mini is a Professor of Medical Oncology at the School of Human Health Sciences and the Director of the Specialty School of Medical Oncology, University of Florence (Italy). He is the Director of the Clinical Program on 'Gastrointestinal Cancer Therapeutics'at the Section of Chemotherapy, Careggi University Hospital, Florence. He is also Head of the Laboratory of Anticancer Chemotherapy at the Department of Health Sciences, University of Florence.

Dr. Mini achieved his M.D. in 1977 and his Ph.D. in 1988 at the University of Florence. He completed his post-graduate training at Yale University School of Medicine (Departments of Pharmacology and Medicine) in the USA. He later became a Lecturer in Pharmacology at the Universities of Siena and Ferrara in Italy. He became an Associate Professor of Pharmacology in the Department of Pharmacology, School of Medicine at the University of Florence in 1992, and Professor of Pharmacology at the School of Medicine (University of Florence) in 2001. In recognition of his achievements, Dr. Mini received the Leukemia Society of America Special Fellow Award in 1982, the Lady Tata Memorial Trust Award and the Alberico Benedicenti Italian Society of Pharmacology Special Mention Award in 1988. Currently, he is a member of the Steering Committee of the European Organization for Research and Treatment of Cancer (EORTC), Pan-European Trials in Adjuvant Colon Cancer (PETACC), and is the Chairman of the Cancer Section of the International Society of Chemotherapy. He is the co-editor of the {Journal of Chemotherapy}. He was also a Visiting Professor at Yale in 2010.

Dr. Mini has authored more than 100 scientific publications. His research interests comprise the mechanisms of tumor drug resistance, in particular to antimetabolites and metal-based drugs, cancer pharmacogenomics and pharmacogenetics, and controlled clinical trials in gastrointestinal cancers.

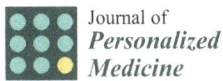

Editorial

Special Issue: "Gastrointestinal Cancers and Personalized Medicine"

Stefania Nobili [1,2,*] and Enrico Mini [3,4]

1. Department of Neurosciences, Imaging and Clinical Sciences, "G. d'Annunzio" University of Chieti-Pescara, 66100 Chieti, Italy
2. Center for Advanced Studies and Technology (CAST), "G. d'Annunzio" University of Chieti-Pescara, 66100 Chieti, Italy
3. Department of Health Sciences, University of Florence, 50139 Florence, Italy; enrico.mini@unifi.it
4. DENOTHE Excellence Center, University of Florence, 50139 Florence, Italy
* Correspondence: stefania.nobili@unich.it

Gastrointestinal cancers represent more than 25% of all diagnosed cancers and more than 36% of cancer-related deaths worldwide [1]. Unfortunately, screening strategies are still limited. They are, in fact, available only for colorectal, gastric and esophageal cancers [2]. However, despite these early diagnostic opportunities, gastrointestinal cancers, including pancreatic, hepatobiliary, small bowel carcinomas and other uncommon cancers, such as anal canal cancer, neuroendocrine tumors of the gastrointestinal tract, primary gastric and intestinal lymphomas, and gastrointestinal stromal tumors (GISTs), are frequently diagnosed at an advanced stage, when treatment options are limited and cure is not possible. Moreover, a very high percentage of patients, about 50%, diagnosed with early potentially curable gastrointestinal cancers, will develop recurrent disease despite surgery, radiation therapy, and pharmacological treatment during the course of the disease [3]. Taken together, these conditions are responsible for poor prognosis in these tumors. Thus, despite current available knowledge on molecular determinants involved in the initiation and progression of cancer [4], there is an urgent clinical need to further improve our biological knowledge of gastrointestinal evolutionary processes toward increased dysregulation, heterogeneity, and the escape from immunosurveillance as well as from pharmacological treatment control [5,6].

Such complex processes substantially involve all types of molecules (e.g., nucleic acids, proteins, metabolites) and involve several cell types, such as transformed epithelial or mesenchymal cells, or other tumor microenvironment cells, including immune cells.

The development and availability of the newest biotechnologies that add knowledge to the field of cancer research strongly contribute to new cancer achievements aimed at discovering and validating novel molecular biomarkers predictive of prognosis and drug response (efficacy/toxicity) in gastrointestinal cancers. A number of cancer biomarkers, mainly represented by somatic alterations in tumor cells (e.g., in the *RAS*, *RAF*, *MMR*, *HER-2* and *KIT* genes), have been identified and validated as clinically useful biomarkers to predict patient prognosis and drug response in gastrointestinal cancers such as colorectal cancer, gastric cancer and GISTs, thus directly contributing to therapeutic decisions.

However, due to the high level of tumor heterogeneity, not only among patients but also among tumor sites in the same patient, the possibility of employing effective personalized medicine for all patients still represents a relevant challenge. Currently, a plethora of potential biomarkers predictive of prognosis or drug response have been suggested [7]. Their detection in tissue and/or in bio-fluidic samples has the potential to improve clinical oncology practice.

In addition, a pharmacogenetic approach, represented by the analysis of germline polymorphisms in genes that play a main role in the ADME of anticancer drugs, has also been progressively introduced into clinical practice for the prediction of the risk of toxicity

Citation: Nobili, S.; Mini, E. Special Issue: "Gastrointestinal Cancers and Personalized Medicine". *J. Pers. Med.* **2022**, *12*, 338. https://doi.org/10.3390/jpm12030338

Received: 21 February 2022
Accepted: 22 February 2022
Published: 24 February 2022

Publisher's Note: MDPI stays neutral with regard to jurisdictional claims in published maps and institutional affiliations.

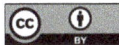

Copyright: © 2022 by the authors. Licensee MDPI, Basel, Switzerland. This article is an open access article distributed under the terms and conditions of the Creative Commons Attribution (CC BY) license (https://creativecommons.org/licenses/by/4.0/).

related to these drugs. However, few polymorphisms in pharmacogenes have been shown to be responsible for drug toxicity. Thus, this aspect still represents a major issue in cancer care.

This Special Issue is designed to provide information on new biomarker research in the area of gastrointestinal tumors that could be useful for innovative personalized management and precision medicine modalities for individualized care.

Gastrointestinal cancers are often diagnosed at advanced stages when therapeutic options are limited. Liquid biopsy, a non-invasive procedure, widely investigated in recent years and already applied to monitor cancer progression and drug resistance, mainly in lung cancer, could also be successfully used to diagnose cancers at early stages. Liquid biopsy, usually performed in blood serum, could be obtained by several different body fluids [8]. Among gastrointestinal cancers, pancreatic cancer could greatly benefit from this opportunity. In fact, although it is only the 12th most common cancer, it is the 6th most common cause of cancer death [1]. Thus, it would be crucial to identify a strategy able to diagnose pancreatic cancer in advance, before tumor development. The incidence of pancreatic cysts is about 2% in adults and neoplastic cysts account for 10–15% of all pancreatic cystic lesions. Although their risk to change in malignant lesions is low, if this occurs, the patient prognosis will be very poor [9].

Hermoso-Durán et al. [10] investigated cyst liquid samples from patients, and the proteomic differences between pancreatic benign and premalignant cysts. To perform such an evaluation the authors used an approach previously used on serum or plasma, named "thermal liquid biopsy" (TLB), which they adapted to cyst liquid samples. Based on the TLB thermograms, cyst profiles were clustered according to their clinical assessment. The authors also elaborated a new TLB serum score based on the specific parameters reflecting differences between cysts. Results were encouraging although the number of analyzed samples was small. The availability of a dedicated TLB as a diagnostic tool for serum samples from patients with pancreatic cysts of which the nature is unknown could represent a relevant advantage in the diagnosis of premalignant lesions of pancreatic cancer.

The prognosis of patients affected by colorectal cancer, one of the most incident and lethal cancers worldwide [1], is highly variable, mainly dependent on the stage at diagnosis. Through the years, many efforts have been made to identify and validate molecular biomarkers predictive of prognosis and/or drug response in this neoplasm. In recent years, interesting examples of predictors of prognosis concern the colorectal cancer molecular subtypes that have been obtained by unsupervised transcriptomic approaches, i.e., consensus colorectal cancer molecular subtypes (CMSs) [11] and colorectal cancer intrinsic subtypes (CRIS) [12]. However, the clinical utility of such classifications for the single patient has yet to be established. Potential biomarkers predictive of response to adjuvant chemotherapy in the early colorectal cancer stages (i.e., stage II-III) have been suggested, for instance from validated transcriptomic [13–15] or genetic [16] analyses. However, to date, biomarkers predictive of drug response represented by actionable oncogenic drivers (i.e., *RAS* wild-type and MSI-H status for anti-EGFR and anti-PD-1 monoclonal antibodies, *BRAF* V600E mutations, *NTRK* gene fusions and more recently *KRAS* G12C mutations for targeted agents) are used only in the metastatic setting [17].

In this framework, the review of Del Buono et al. [18] contextualized the role of the DNA mismatch repair (MMR) system in colorectal cancer precision medicine. Today, the knowledge of the MSI status provides several advantages by satisfying a number of clinical queries. In fact, MSI, due to an impaired MMR system, plays a role in the inherited predisposition to gastrointestinal cancers, and identifies a subset of colorectal cancer patients who show a substantial better prognosis and who do not obtain an advantage from adjuvant chemotherapy (i.e., low-risk stage II patients). More recently, MSI has become a key biomarker for the treatment of several tumors, including colorectal cancer, with immune checkpoint inhibitors. Thus, the evaluation of MMR/MSI is becoming part of standard care in colorectal cancer, as recommended by major oncological international societies [17].

Overall, therapeutic options in colorectal cancer are related to the cancer stage and, as mentioned above, differ from metastatic and nonmetastatic settings. Stage I and low-risk stage II patients are treated with surgery alone. High-risk stage II, stage III and stage IV (oligometastatic disease) patients are instead treated with pharmacological therapy in addition to surgery, with positive results. However, neoplastic progression due to additional dysregulated molecular events occurs in a substantial percentage of patients, limiting the efficacy of the available drugs administered as adjuvant or neoadjuvant therapies. This occurrence stimulates the search for biomarkers able to predict colorectal cancer prognosis in order to plan preventative pharmacological strategies for patients at high risk of disease progression as well as biomarkers predictive of drug response, in order to avoid the administration of inactive drugs to resistant patients. Immunoscore is a further example of tumor biomarker able to predict disease prognosis in early-stage colorectal cancer [19]. Instead, tumor mutational burden is not yet a recommended biomarker for the prediction of pembrolizumab efficacy in colorectal cancer due to the limited data available in this patient population [17].

The study of Rhyner Agocs et al. [20] evaluated the predictive role of the expression of the lymphocyte-activation gene 3 (LAG-3) in the outcome of 143 stage II colon cancer. LAG-3 is an inhibitory immune-related molecule mainly expressed on T cells, but also on B cells and dendritic cells. LAG-3 may synergize with the PD-1/PD-L1 pathway and is closely related to CD4. The upregulation of LAG-3 on immune cells downregulates T cell expansion and cytokine secretion, and thus contributes to an immunosuppressive microenvironment. In particular, the presence of LAG-3 was evaluated by immunohistochemistry in formalin-fixed paraffin-embedded (FFPE) tissues on tumor-infiltrating lymphocytes (TILs) in the tumor center and tumor front to assess its impact on the survival of stage II colon cancer patients. The authors found no correlations between LAG-3 expression and clinical/pathological characteristics, although they observed a higher percentage of MMR-deficient colon cancers when LAG-3-positive TILS were present. In relation to the primary study end-point, i.e., disease-free survival, the authors found a significant association between the presence of LAG-3 in the tumor front and prolonged disease-free survival. This significant correlation was maintained even when only MMR-proficient colon cancer, (i.e., the majority of the analyzed tumors), were considered. Moreover, in this case, such a correlation was limited to TILs localized at the tumor front. Thus, this manuscript identified LAG-3 as a biomarker potentially useful in predicting patient prognosis in stage II colon cancer, including MMR-proficient tumors.

Similarly, Peyravian et al. [21] analyzed a panel of candidate genes (i.e., 20 genes) whose expression was potentially involved in the development of lymph node metastases in 100 colorectal cancer patients. The selected genes were chosen according to their role in key cancer processes such as carcinogenesis, tumor growth, tumor invasion and metastasis. Overall, about 60% of patients initially diagnosed as stage I-III, were lymph nodes negative. Hierarchical clustering analysis showed that *VANGL1*, *PCSK7*, and *ANXA3* genes were the most expressed among the study genes at mRNA level in the majority of colorectal cancer samples. However, only *VANGL1* was shown to significantly vary between lymph node-negative and -positive patients. The mRNA expression levels of *VANGL1* were also confirmed at protein level. The study also provided associations between two other study genes, *NOTCH1* and *ILR2B*, and overall survival. In particular, the high expression of *NOTCH1* and the low expression of *ILR2B* were associated with prolonged overall survival.

In metastatic colorectal cancer, Taghizadeh et al. [22] provided a molecular profile of a real-world cohort of drug refractory patients for whom no further standard treatment option was available. The molecular profile was performed by a precision medicine platform developed at the author's institution, i.e., the Comprehensive Cancer Centre of the Medical University of Vienna. Based on the biomolecular characteristics of tumors, this study was aimed at providing information on potential further options of targeted therapy. Overall, by exploiting next-generation sequencing panels of mutation hotspots, microsatellite instability testing, and immunohistochemistry, 60 metastatic colorectal cancer samples were characterized. The analysis revealed 166 mutations in 53 patients, the five most frequent being *TP53, KRAS, APC, PIK3CA*, and *PTEN*. All patients had previously received cytotoxic chemotherapy combined with anti-EGFR or anti-VEGF(R) monoclonal antibodies. The study showed that, in 47% of patients, a molecularly targeted therapy could be recommended whereas the remaining were not suitable for targeted therapy due to the lack of actionable molecular targets. Overall, 20% of the study patients underwent the recommended targeted therapy. In particular, pembrolizumab was offered to four MSI-H patients, consequently obtaining control of disease in all patients and objective response in 75%. Stable disease was observed in two further patients treated with everolimus combined with raltitrexed, and with trastuzumab combined with lapatinib, respectively, according to their specific immunohistochemical and mutational characteristics (i.e., strong m-TOR expression associated with the loss of PTEN and HER2+ overexpression, respectively). Overall, this study highlights how at least a portion of heavily pretreated patients without further standard treatment options may benefit from a molecular-based treatment approach.

Interestingly, by a rationale based on the role that the immune response and inflammation play in tumor growth and in the metastatic process, Fülöp et al. [23] evaluated the prognostic impact of the neutrophil-to-lymphocyte and lymphocyte-to-monocyte ratios (i.e., NLR and LMR) in over 1000 rectal cancer patients. The overall survival was significantly associated with increased NLR and decreased LMR, and no relationship was found between the study ratios and tumor stage, thus potentially suggesting that these markers are independent from cancer stage, even if this occurrence is controversial [24]. Moreover, NLR and LMR were also found to predict response to the neoadjuvant chemoradiotherapy to which patients underwent. In particular, the identification of a cut-off for NLR value (i.e., ≥ 3.11) allowed the authors to discriminate between chemoradiotherapy responsive and non-responsive rectal cancer patients, although the responsive ones had a low chance of sphincter preservation, or to obtain a complete total mesorectal excision. Although the study ratios may also be affected by factors independent of the neoplastic disease, these data warrant attention due to the high number of patients included in this analysis and deserve further investigation.

Oxaliplatin, widely used in the treatment of gastrointestinal cancers, is a highly neurotoxic agent. Acute or chronic peripheral neuropathy develops in about 90% and 40% of patients, respectively, and the latter form may strongly affect the quality of life of patients and cancer survivors. Unfortunately, to date, no remedy or antidote is available to reverse this side effect. Thus, it would be very important to identify patients susceptible to develop peripheral neuropathy before starting the oxaliplatin treatment, even though, despite the efforts of many researchers, no predictive biomarker has yet been identified.

The review of Velasco et al. [25] discusses the status of the art of strategies that may be implemented pre-emptively to evaluate the risk of developing neurotoxicity. In particular, neurological monitoring through the evaluation of neurophysiological signs of oxaliplatin-induced neuropathy may be performed by mechanical strategies (e.g., nerve conduction tests, electromyography). However, this procedure is not part of the common clinical practice. Less invasive blood biomarkers have also been widely investigated. Genetic biomarkers, mainly represented by single-nucleotide polymorphisms in genes encoding detoxification enzymes (e.g., proteins belonging to the glutathione detoxification system), drug transporters (e.g., ATP binding proteins), proteins involved in the mechanism of action of oxaliplatin, as well as proteins implicated in neuronal functions, have drawn attention. In addition, proteins released in blood when nerve damage occurs (e.g., the protein neurofilament light chain (NfL) and nerve growth factor (NGF)) have also been suggested as predictive biomarkers of neurotoxicity. Neuroimaging strategies have also been studied as potential tools for the early detection of neurotoxicity onset.

Overall, the manuscripts included in this Special Issue highlight the need to identify and validate molecular biomarkers predictive of prognosis and drug response in gastrointestinal cancers. To satisfy this goal, biomarkers identified in retrospective studies will need to be validated in large-scale prospective clinical trials. Moreover, the availability of new and highly predictive biomarkers implies that the discovery of new anticancer drugs, specifically inhibiting these targets, can be accomplished to effectively treat patients who are potentially unresponsive to standard therapies.

Conflicts of Interest: The authors declare no conflict of interest.

References

1. Sung, H.; Ferlay, J.; Siegel, R.L.; Laversanne, M.; Soerjomataram, I.; Jemal, A.; Bray, F. Global Cancer Statistics 2020: GLOBOCAN Estimates of Incidence and Mortality Worldwide for 36 Cancers in 185 Countries. *CA Cancer J. Clin.* **2021**, *71*, 209–249. [CrossRef]
2. Baraniskin, A.; Van Laethem, J.L.; Wyrwicz, L.; Guller, U.; Wasan, H.S.; Matysiak-Budnik, T.; Gruenberger, T.; Ducreux, M.; Carneiro, F.; Van Cutsem, E.; et al. Clinical relevance of molecular diagnostics in gastrointestinal (GI) cancer: European Society of Digestive Oncology (ESDO) expert discussion and recommendations from the 17th European Society for Medical Oncology (ESMO)/World Congress on Gastrointestinal Cancer, Barcelona. *Eur. J. Cancer* **2017**, *86*, 305–317. [CrossRef]
3. Sonnenberg, W.R. Gastrointestinal Malignancies. *Prim. Care* **2017**, *44*, 721–732. [CrossRef]
4. Vogelstein, B.; Papadopoulos, N.; Velculescu, V.E.; Zhou, S.; Diaz, L.A., Jr.; Kinzler, K.W. Cancer genome landscapes. *Science* **2013**, *339*, 1546–1558. [CrossRef]
5. Alison, M.R. The cellular origins of cancer with particular reference to the gastrointestinal tract. *Int. J. Exp. Pathol.* **2020**, *101*, 132–151. [CrossRef]
6. Koessler, T.; Alsina, M.; Arnold, D.; Ben-Aharon, I.; Lutz, M.P.; Obermannova, R.; Peeters, M.; Sclafani, F.; Smyth, E.; Valle, J.W.; et al. Highlights from ASCO-GI 2021 from EORTC Gastrointestinal tract cancer group. *Br. J. Cancer* **2021**, *125*, 911–919. [CrossRef]
7. Pal, M.; Muinao, T.; Boruah, H.P.D.; Mahindroo, N. Current advances in prognostic and diagnostic biomarkers for solid cancers: Detection techniques and future challenges. *Biomed. Pharmacother.* **2022**, *146*, 112488. [CrossRef]
8. Santos, V.; Freitas, C.; Fernandes, M.G.; Sousa, C.; Reboredo, C.; Cruz-Martins, N.; Mosquera, J.; Hespanhol, V.; Campelo, R. Liquid biopsy: The value of different bodily fluids. *Biomark. Med.* **2022**, *16*, 127–145. [CrossRef]
9. Buerlein, R.C.D.; Shami, V.M. Management of pancreatic cysts and guidelines: What the gastroenterologist needs to know. *Ther. Adv. Gastrointest. Endosc.* **2021**, *14*, 26317745211045769. [CrossRef]
10. Hermoso-Durán, S.; García-Rayado, G.; Ceballos-Laita, L.; Sostres, C.; Vega, S.; Millastre, J.; Sánchez-Gracia, O.; Ojeda, J.L.; Lanas, Á.; Velázquez-Campoy, A.; et al. Thermal Liquid Biopsy (TLB) Focused on Benign and Premalignant Pancreatic Cyst Diagnosis. *J. Pers. Med.* **2020**, *11*, 25. [CrossRef]
11. Guinney, J.; Dienstmann, R.; Wang, X.; de Reyniès, A.; Schlicker, A.; Soneson, C.; Marisa, L.; Roepman, P.; Nyamundanda, G.; Angelino, P.; et al. The consensus molecular subtypes of colorectal cancer. *Nat. Med.* **2015**, *21*, 1350–1356. [CrossRef]
12. Isella, C.; Brundu, F.; Bellomo, S.E.; Galimi, F.; Zanella, E.; Porporato, R.; Petti, C.; Fiori, A.; Orzan, F.; Senetta, R.; et al. Selective analysis of cancer-cell intrinsic transcriptional traits defines novel clinically relevant subtypes of colorectal cancer. *Nat. Commun.* **2017**, *8*, 15107. [CrossRef]
13. Allen, W.L.; Dunne, P.D.; McDade, S.; Scanlon, E.; Loughrey, M.; Coleman, H.; McCann, C.; McLaughlin, K.; Nemeth, Z.; Syed, N.; et al. Transcriptional subtyping and CD8 immunohistochemistry identifies poor prognosis stage II/III colorectal cancer patients who benefit from adjuvant chemotherapy. *JCO Precis. Oncol.* **2018**, *2018*, PO.17.00241. [CrossRef]
14. Mini, E.; Lapucci, A.; Perrone, G.; D'Aurizio, R.; Napoli, C.; Brugia, M.; Landini, I.; Tassi, R.; Picariello, L.; Simi, L.; et al. RNA sequencing reveals PNN and KCNQ1OT1 as predictive biomarkers of clinical outcome in stage III colorectal cancer patients treated with adjuvant chemotherapy. *Int. J. Cancer* **2019**, *145*, 2580–2593. [CrossRef]
15. Lapucci, A.; Perrone, G.; Di Paolo, A.; Napoli, C.; Landini, I.; Roviello, G.; Calosi, L.; Naccarato, A.G.; Falcone, A.; Bani, D.; et al. *PNN* and *KCNQ1OT1* Can Predict the Efficacy of Adjuvant Fluoropyrimidine-Based Chemotherapy in Colorectal Cancer Patients. *Oncol. Res.* **2021**, *28*, 631–644. [CrossRef]
16. Park, H.A.; Seibold, P.; Edelmann, D.; Benner, A.; Canzian, F.; Alwers, E.; Jansen, L.; Schneider, M.; Hoffmeister, M.; Brenner, H.; et al. Validation of Genetic Markers Associated with Survival in Colorectal Cancer Patients Treated with Oxaliplatin-Based Chemotherapy. *Cancer Epidemiol. Biomark. Prev.* **2022**, *31*, 352–361. [CrossRef]
17. NCCN. Clinical Practice Guidelines in Oncology—Colon Cancer—V. 3.2021. Available online: https://www.nccn.org/professionals/physician_gls/pdf/colon.pdf (accessed on 14 February 2022).
18. Dal Buono, A.; Gaiani, F.; Poliani, L.; Correale, C.; Laghi, L. Defects in MMR Genes as a Seminal Example of Personalized Medicine: From Diagnosis to Therapy. *J. Pers. Med.* **2021**, *11*, 1333. [CrossRef]
19. Mini, E.; Landini, I.; Di Paolo, A.; Ravegnini, G.; Saponara, S.; Frosini, M.; Lapucci, A.; Nobili, S. Predictive 'Omic' biomarkers of drug response: Colorectal cancer as a model. In *Anti-Angiogenic Drugs as Chemosensitizers in Cancer Therapy*; Morbidelli, L., Ed.; Cancer Sensitizing Agents for Chemotherapy Series; Elsevier Inc.: Academic Press, London, UK, 2022; Volume 18, pp. 199–240. [CrossRef]
20. Rhyner Agocs, G.; Assarzadegan, N.; Kirsch, R.; Dawson, H.; Galván, J.A.; Lugli, A.; Zlobec, I.; Berger, M.D. LAG-3 Expression Predicts Outcome in Stage II Colon Cancer. *J. Pers. Med.* **2021**, *11*, 749. [CrossRef]
21. Peyravian, N.; Nobili, S.; Pezeshkian, Z.; Olfatifar, M.; Moradi, A.; Baghaei, K.; Anaraki, F.; Nazari, K.; Asadzadeh Aghdaei, H.; Zali, M.R.; et al. Increased Expression of *VANGL1* is Predictive of Lymph Node Metastasis in Colorectal Cancer: Results from a 20-Gene Expression Signature. *J. Pers. Med.* **2021**, *11*, 126. [CrossRef]

22. Taghizadeh, H.; Mader, R.M.; Müllauer, L.; Erhart, F.; Kautzky-Willer, A.; Prager, G.W. Precision Medicine for the Management of Therapy Refractory Colorectal Cancer. *J. Pers. Med.* **2020**, *10*, 272. [CrossRef]
23. Fülöp, Z.Z.; Gurzu, S.; Fülöp, R.L.; Bara, T., Jr.; Tímár, J.; Drágus, E.; Jung, I. Prognostic Impact of the Neutrophil-to-Lymphocyte and Lymphocyte-to-Monocyte Ratio.; in Patients with Rectal Cancer: A Retrospective Study of 1052 Patients. *J. Pers. Med.* **2020**, *10*, 173. [CrossRef]
24. Howard, R.; Kanetsky, P.A.; Egan, K.M. Exploring the prognostic value of the neutrophil-to-lymphocyte ratio in cancer. *Sci. Rep.* **2019**, *9*, 19673. [CrossRef]
25. Velasco, R.; Alemany, M.; Villagrán, M.; Argyriou, A.A. Predictive Biomarkers of Oxaliplatin-Induced Peripheral Neurotoxicity. *J. Pers. Med.* **2021**, *11*, 669. [CrossRef]

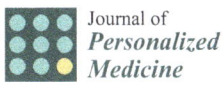

Article

Thermal Liquid Biopsy (TLB) Focused on Benign and Premalignant Pancreatic Cyst Diagnosis

Sonia Hermoso-Durán [1,2,†], Guillermo García-Rayado [1,3,4,†], Laura Ceballos-Laita [1,2], Carlos Sostres [1,3,4], Sonia Vega [2], Judith Millastre [1,3], Oscar Sánchez-Gracia [5], Jorge L. Ojeda [6], Ángel Lanas [1,3,4,7], Adrián Velázquez-Campoy [1,2,4,8,9,*] and Olga Abian [1,2,4,8,10,*]

1. Instituto de Investigación Sanitaria Aragón (IIS Aragón), 50009 Zaragoza, Spain; shermosod@gmail.com (S.H.-D.); guillermogarcia7@hotmail.com (G.G.-R.); ceballos.laita@gmail.com (L.C.-L.); carlossostres@gmail.com (C.S.); millastrej@gmail.com (J.M.); alanas@unizar.es (Á.L.)
2. Joint Units IQFR-CSIC-BIFI, and GBsC-CSIC-BIFI, Institute of Biocomputation and Physics of Complex Systems (BIFI), Universidad de Zaragoza, 50018 Zaragoza, Spain; svega@bifi.es
3. Servicio de Digestivo, Hospital Clínico Universitario Lozano Blesa (HCULB), 50009 Zaragoza, Spain
4. Centro de Investigación Biomédica en Red en el Área Temática de Enfermedades Hepáticas y Digestivas (CIBERehd), 28029 Madrid, Spain
5. SOTER BioAnalytics, Enrique Val, 50011 Zaragoza, Spain; oscar.sanchez.gracia@gmail.com
6. Department of Statistical Methods, Universidad de Zaragoza, 50009 Zaragoza, Spain; jojeda@unizar.es
7. Department of Medicine, University of Zaragoza, 50009 Zaragoza, Spain
8. Fundación ARAID, Gobierno de Aragón, 50009 Zaragoza, Spain
9. Departamento de Bioquímica y Biología Molecular y Celular, Universidad de Zaragoza, 50009 Zaragoza, Spain
10. Instituto Aragonés de Ciencias de la Salud (IACS), 50009 Zaragoza, Spain
* Correspondence: adrianvc@unizar.es (A.V.-C.); oabifra@unizar.es (O.A.); Tel.: +34-976-762996 (A.V.-C.); +34-876-555417 (O.A.)
† S.H.-D. and G.G.-R. contributed equally to this work and are both first authors of the manuscript.

Abstract: Background: Current efforts in the identification of new biomarkers are directed towards an accurate differentiation between benign and premalignant cysts. Thermal Liquid Biopsy (TLB) has been previously applied to inflammatory and tumor diseases and could offer an interesting point of view in this type of pathology. Methods: In this work, twenty patients (12 males and 8 females, average ages 62) diagnosed with a pancreatic cyst benign (10) and premalignant (10) cyst lesions were recruited, and biological samples were obtained during the endoscopic ultrasonography procedure. Results: Proteomic content of cyst liquid samples was studied and several common proteins in the different groups were identified. TLB cyst liquid profiles reflected protein content. Also, TLB serum score was able to discriminate between healthy and cysts patients (71% sensitivity and 98% specificity) and between benign and premalignant cysts (75% sensitivity and 67% specificity). Conclusions: TLB analysis of plasmatic serum sample, a quick, simple and non-invasive technique that can be easily implemented, reports valuable information on the observed pancreatic lesion. These preliminary results set the basis for a larger study to refine TLB serum score and move closer to the clinical application of TLB providing useful information to the gastroenterologist during patient diagnosis.

Keywords: pancreatic cysts; thermal liquid biopsy; differential scanning calorimetry; diagnosis; generalized linear models

1. Introduction

During recent years, the detection of pancreatic cysts has become more frequent due to improvements in abdominal imaging techniques. The incidence of this pathology is approximately 2% in the adult population [1]. Computed tomography (CT) scans are reported detection between 1.2% and 2.6%, and magnetic resonance imaging (MRI) has even a higher detection capability, ranging between 13.5% and 19.9% [1,2]. The management of

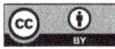

these incidentally detected pancreatic cysts is still a challenge, because, even though the risk of being malignant is low, the prognosis in case of pancreatic adenocarcinoma and intraductal papillary mucinous neoplasms- (IPMN)-related pancreatic adenocarcinoma is very poor and has not improved recently [3]. Thus, distinguishing between benign and malignant cysts is difficult, and very often requires surgical intervention with considerable morbidity and mortality. Since 2005, some guidelines have been published and updated: the American Society for Gastrointestinal Endoscopy [4], international consensus guidelines by the International Association of Pancreatology (Sendai guidelines) [5], the American College of Gastroenterology [6], and the International Association of Pancreatology (Fukuoka guidelines) [7,8]. More recently, The European Study Group on Cystic Tumors of the Pancreas published an update, replacing the 2013 European Consensus Statement Guidelines [9].

From a clinical point of view, the classification according to the prognosis of the lesion is: (1) cysts with malignant potential (mucinous), (2) cysts without malignant potential, and (3) malignancies. However, most studies provide a description of biomarkers for differentiating the mucinous and non-mucinous type of cysts. The non-mucinous group comprises serous cystadenomas (SCAs) (the most common type), pancreatic pseudocysts (PCs), and a variety of rare cysts (benign epithelial, lymphoepithelial, congenital, and squamoid cysts). Most are found incidentally and none of them represents a risk for becoming malignant [10]. On the contrary, the mucinous group, including mucinous cystic neoplasms (MCNs) and IPMNs, constitutes the majority of neoplastic premalignant cysts identified in the pancreas, and a precise diagnosis technique would be vital for the management of patients [11]. The development of techniques with greater pre-surgical diagnostic precision would make it possible to avoid the morbidity and mortality associated with a high-risk intervention when it is not strictly necessary, as well as reduce the healthcare overload derived from unnecessary outpatient follow-up in cystic lesions without the potential for malignancy.

Cystic fluid markers become especially relevant when transabdominal ultrasonography, CT or MRI are inconclusive. In these cases, it is necessary to employ another risk predictor to indicate surgery as the most appropriate treatment given the estimated risk.

The presence of amylase at high concentration in cyst fluid indicates that there is a communication between the cyst and the ductal system. This occurs in both pseudocysts and IPMN lesions. When amylase levels are lower than 250 U/L, communication with the conduct can be discarded, with a specificity of 98% [12]. However, amylase value alone is not enough to differentiate between mucinous/non-mucinous or MCN/IPMN, which is important from the point of view of patient management, in deciding whether surgical resection or cyst time-monitoring is recommended [13]. A previous episode of pancreatitis can be of help in distinguishing a pseudocyst from an IPMN lesion (occasionally related to pancreatitis) [14].

Carcinoembryonic antigen (CEA) is also employed as a biomarker. This is a set of highly related glycoproteins involved in cell adhesion, mucin being one of them. It can be used to distinguish between cysts with (MCNs and IPMNs) and without (SCAs and PCs) mucinous epithelium [10]. The major inconvenience of CEA is the absence of an appropriate cutoff value [12]. The current accepted value to classify a cyst as mucinous is CEA > 192 ng/mL [15].

In order to improve diagnosis, studies related to the identification of new biomarkers in cystic fluid or serum have been recently reported [16–21].

In 2007 Chaires et al. [22] described the application of differential scanning calorimetry (DSC) in diagnosis using plasma/serum samples from cancer patients. Since then, many studies have confirmed the potential clinical use of this technique, not only applied to plasma/serum [23–30], but also to other biological human samples such as cerebrospinal fluid [31,32]. In 2018 our group coined the name "thermal liquid biopsy" (TLB) for DSC applied to cancer diagnosis and cancer patient's treatment monitoring [33,34]. The TLB thermogram reports the global denaturation profile for all the proteins present in the serum/plasma sample and the influence of potential interactions between blood plasma proteins and metabolites, therefore reflecting any alteration induced by a certain disease. As in the case of plasma or serum, cystic fluid is also composed of a mixture of proteins and TLB may also be applied as a clinical diagnosis tool. In this work, the potential of TLB as a clinical biomarker for cyst classification has been pursued. In this pilot study, 20 cyst fluid samples were analyzed and their TLB cyst profiles were obtained, with the purpose of finding a correlation between the TLB thermogram and the type of cyst. The proteomic analysis also allowed a description of the more abundant proteins in the cyst fluid, as well as the post-translational modifications present in those proteins. TLB was also applied to serum samples in some of the patients, and TLB serum profile differences between groups was studied to try to determine whether or not differences observed in cyst fluid TLB correlated with serum TLB. This would be extremely important because, in case cyst features are reflected in certain serum alterations, a simple and risk-free plasma/serum TLB analysis could be employed for cyst diagnosis/classification. Despite the low number of samples considered in this pilot study, different patterns in cyst fluid and plasma from patients with pathology could be observed.

2. Materials and Methods

2.1. Subjects and Samples

Cyst liquid and serum samples from patients with cystic lesions in the pancreas detected by transabdominal ultrasonography or CT or MRI were referred to the Department of Digestive Endoscopy at the Hospital Clínico Universitario Lozano Blesa (HCULB), Zaragoza, Spain, between January 2016 and September 2018. The procedure was in accordance with the recommendations of the local ethics committee and all patients gave their informed consent. Pancreatic cystic fluids were collected by EUS-guided fine needle aspiration (FNA). The EUS-FNA procedure was performed with an Olympus® 140 curvilinear echo-endoscope. Boston Scientific™ Expect® 19 or 22-gauge needles were used depending on the cystic endosonographic features. We noted the characteristics of the aspirated cystic fluid: volume, color, and viscosity. The majority of the fluid was examined by the same cytopathologist for every patient and the rest (at least 1 mL Eppendorf for each patient) was collected for detection of biochemical markers, DSC measurements, and proteomic studies described in this manuscript. The collected cystic fluid samples were then stored at $-80\,^\circ$C until they were prepared for analysis.

Serum samples from healthy subjects as control group (HC) consisted of 85 serum samples from Spanish Caucasian subjects, apparently cancer-free, from the FISABIO (Fundación para el Fomento de la Investigacion Sanitaria y Biomedica de la Comunitat Valenciana) biobank with a homogeneous distribution, including gender (53% men and 47% women), with an average age of 45.2 ± 14.2.

2.2. Thermal Liquid Biopsy (TLB) Profile Determination

DSC thermograms were measured using a high-sensitivity differential scanning VP-DSC microcalorimeter (MicroCal, Malvern-Panalytical, Malvern, UK). Cystic liquid samples, serum samples, and reference solutions were properly degassed and carefully loaded into the cells to avoid bubble formation. The baseline of the instrument was routinely recorded before the experiments. Experiments were performed in cystic liquid samples (diluted 1:10 in phosphate buffered saline, PBS) and serum samples (diluted 1:25 in PBS) at a scanning rate of $1\,^\circ$C/min. Thermograms were baseline-corrected and analyzed using software developed in our laboratory implemented in Origin 7 (OriginLab, Northampton, MA, USA).

2.3. Data Analysis

We have developed a phenomenological model in which the TLB serum thermogram is deconvoluted into several individual transitions, modeling each individual transition by the logistic peak or Hubbert function [30,33]. This model has been successfully applied in the analysis of serum samples from melanoma and gastric and lung cancer patients [30,34,35].

From this multiparametric analysis, a TLB serum score (between 0 and 1) can be calculated reporting the level of alterations in plasma (TLB serum score < 0.5, absence of alterations; TLB serum score > 0.5, presence of alterations).

The Kolmogorov-Smirnov test was performed to assess the normal distribution of the variables. Medians between two independent groups were compared with the Wilcoxon test, in non-normal distributions. Averages between two independent groups were compared with the *t*-test, in normal distributions.

2.4. Protein Sample Preparation and Protein Identification and Quantification by Mass Spectrometry

Protein concentration: Measured by Bradford protein assay (Bio-Rad, Madrid, Spain) using purified bovine serum albumin (BSA) (10 mg/mL, New England BioLabs, EVRY cedex, France) in PBS as standard. Absorbance at 595 nm of two dilutions from each serum sample was measured in triplicate in a Synergy HT multimode microplate reader (BioTek Instruments, Winooski, VT, USA).

In solution digestion: Samples were evaporated and resuspended in 10 µL of denaturing buffer (6 M urea, 100 mM Tris buffer pH 7.8). Next, cysteines were reduced with 1.5 µL DTT (200 mM) for 30 min at 37 °C and alkylated with 6 µL of iodoacetamide (200 mM) for 30 min in the dark. Unreacted iodoacetamide was consumed adding 6 µL of the reducing agent (200 mM DTT) for 30 min at room temperature. Samples were diluted with 50 mM ammonium bicarbonate to a urea final concentration lower than 1 M. Trypsin digestion (Gold Trypsin, Promega, Madison, WI, USA) was carried out overnight at 37 °C at a 1:20 enzyme/protein ratio. Reaction was stopped adding concentrated formic acid (Merck KGaA, Darmstadt, Germany). Samples were evaporated, resuspended in 2% acetonitrile (ACN), 0.1% formic acid, and filtered through 0.45 µm filters.

Protein identification by LC-ESI-MS/MS: Protein identification was performed on a nano-LC 2D system (LC 425, Eksigent Ekspert TM, Dublin, CA, USA) coupled to a hybrid triple quadrupole/linear ion trap mass spectrometer (4000 QTRAP, Sciex, Foster City, CA, USA). On-line pre-concentration and desalting of samples was performed using a C18 trap cartridge (Luna® 0.3 mm id, 20 mm, 5 µm particle size, Phenomenex, CA, USA) at 10 µL/min for 5 min. Peptide separation was performed using a C18 column (Gemini® 0.3 mm id, 150 mm, 3 µm particle size, Phenomenex, CA, USA), at 5 µL/min of flow rate. Column was maintained at 35 °C. The elution gradient was from 5 to 35% ACN (0.1% formic acid) in 90 min. The mass spectrometer was interfaced with an ESI source (Turbo V™) using a 25 µm ID hybrid electrode and was operated in the positive ion mode. MS source parameters were as follows: capillary voltage 5000 V, de-clustering potential (DP) 85 V and curtain and ion source gas (Nitrogen) 15 psi. Analyses were performed using an information dependent acquisition (IDA) method with the following steps: single enhanced mass spectra (EMS, 400–1400 m/z) from which the 5 most intense peaks were subjected to an enhanced product ion [EPI (MS/MS)] scan. Protein identification was carried out using the Mascot search engine (Matrix Science; London, UK) and the non-redundant SwissProt database (553,655 sequences; 198,177,566 residues). Search parameters were monoisotopic mass accuracy, peptide mass tolerance ±0.5 Da, fragment mass tolerance ±0.3 Da; one allowed missed cleavage; allowed fixed modification carbamido-methylation (Cys), and variable modification oxidation (Met). Positive identification was assigned with Mascot scores above the threshold level ($p < 0.05$), with at least two identified peptides with a score above homology

Protein SDS electrophoresis: Samples mixed with NuPAGE LDS Sample buffer (Invitrogen), and heated at 95 °C for 4 min, were analysed by sodium dodecyl sulphate–polyacrylamide gel electrophoresis (SDS–PAGE) using 10% acrylamide resolving gels and 4% acrylamide stacking gels (Bio-Rad). The gels were fixed with a mixture of ethanol, acetic acid, and deionized water (40:10:50) for 1 h. After washing in water for 5 min, the gels were stained with Coomassie Brilliant Blue R250 (0.1% in 25% methanol, 10% acetic acid) and de-stained by incubation in 30% acetic acid and 20% methanol. Molecular weights were estimated by comparison with the migration rates of standard proteins (Bio-Rad).

3. Results

3.1. Clinical Sample Description

Patients who underwent endoscopic ultrasonography procedure were included in this work. A total of 20 subjects, 60 and 40% men and women, respectively, with an average age of 62 ± 13 years.

Based on imaging and cytopathology, the pancreatic cysts were classified into different categories (Table 1).

Table 1. Patient Description.

	Type of Cyst						Non-Cyst Malignant Lesions	
	Benign			Pre-Malignant				
	PC ($n = 5$)	WOPN ($n = 3$)	SC ($n = 1$)	LYM ($n = 1$)	IPMN ($n = 7$)	MCN ($n = 1$)	PDAC ($n = 2$)	Total ($n = 20$)
Age (years) *	63 ± 10	62 ± 10	72 ± 0	52 ± 0	72 ± 13	42 ± 0	40 ± 2	62 ± 13
Male/female %	80/20	67/33	100/0	0/100	71/29	0/100	0/100	60/40

* Average ± standard deviation (sd) PC = pseudocyst; WOPN = Walled-off pancreatic necrosis; IPMN = intraductal papillary mucinous neoplasm; SC= Serous Cyst; MCN= Mucinous Cystadenoma; LYM= lymphocele; PDAC= Pancreatic Ductal Adenocarcinoma.

Clinical information of the samples is detailed in Table 2. All the cysts were between 2 and 15 cm in size and they were located in any region in the pancreas. According to clinical data (amylase and CEA concentrations), samples were divided in two groups: benign cysts (PC, WOPN and SC) and premalignant cysts (IPMN and MCN). There are two samples that turned out not to be cysts, but malignant lesions (PDAC).

Table 2. Clinical Cyst Sample Description.

Group	Name	Localization in the Pancreas	Cyst Size (cm)	Amylase (U/L)	CEA (ng/mL)	Final Clinical Diagnosis
Benign Cysts	PC1	Body	5.5	>11,000.0	9.23	Pseudocyst (In Acute Pancreatitis Context)
	PC2	Head	4.1	>11,000.0	64.2	Pseudocyst
	PC3	Head	3.5	5635.0	68.4	Pseudocyst
	PC4	Body	15.0	nd	nd	Pseudocyst (In Acute Pancreatitis Context)
	PC5	Head	3.0	>11,000.0	28.8	Pseudocyst (In Chronic Pancreatitis Context)
	WOPN1	Tail	6.4	>11,000.0	2.4	Walled-off pancreatic necrosis
	WOPN2	Head	10.0	>11,000.0	2.0	Walled-off pancreatic necrosis
	WOPN3	Body	4.0	>11,000.0	50.0	Walled-off pancreatic necrosis
	SC1	Body	5.0	41.0	0.7	Serous Cyst
	LYM	Head	4.9	24.0	0.8	Lymphocele
Pre-Malignant Cysts	IPMN1	Body	2.6	>11,000.0	489.2	Branch duct IPMN
	IPMN2	Head, Body, Tail	2.0	162.0	1488.0	Main duct IPMN
	IPMN3	Head	2.3	>11,000.0	156.0	Branch duct IPMN
	IPMN4	Head	2.5	>11,000.0	556.0	Branch duct IPMN
	IPMN5	Isthmus	3.5	>11,000.0	225.0	Mixed Branch and Main duct IPMN
	IPMN 6	Head	3.0	10.0	392.0	Main Duct IPMN with pancreatic extension
	IPMN 7	Head, Body, Tail	3.5	4.0	>50,000.0	Main Duct IPMN with pancreatic extension
	MCN1	Body	3.3	3401.0	1617.0	Mucinous Cystadenoma
Non-Cyst Malignant Lesions	PDAC 1	Body, Tail	8.0	nd	nd	Pancreatic Ductal Adenocarcinoma
	PDAC 2	Head	0.5	>11,000.0	1192.0	Pancreatic Ductal Adenocarcinoma

nd = not determined: Amylase < 250 U/L, communication with the conduct can be discarded; CEA > 192 ng/mL to classify a cyst as mucinous.

Pancreatic pseudocysts (PC) are pockets of fluid, common sequelae of acute pancreatitis or chronic pancreatitis. PCs are important in terms of management and differentiation from other cystic processes or masses in this region. According to the updated Atlanta classification [36], there are two main groups of mature-well defined fluid collections associated with acute pancreatitis: A/Fluid collections in interstitial edematous pancreatitis (PC), and B/Fluid collections in necrotizing pancreatitis (WOPN). Both PC and WOPN were considered benign cysts. From our PC samples, PC 1 and 4 were in the context of acute pancreatitis, and PC 5 was in the context of chronic pancreatitis. The WOPN cysts had the biggest size, between 3 and 15 cm. Both types of pancreatic collections (PC and WOPN) were amylase positive (above 250 U/L) and CEA negative (below 192 ng/mL).

Serous cysts (SC) are benign neoplasms composed of numerous small cysts that are arrayed in a honeycomb-like formation and most individual cysts are typically <10 mm.

Lymphocele (LYM), also known as cystic lymphangioma, is a rare disease. There are no typical clinical manifestations, and most patients were diagnosed incidentally during imaging or surgery. Therefore, diagnosis is challenging. Surgical resection is still considered as the most effective approach for lymphocele, and prognosis is favorable. In our study, SC and Lym were 5 cm in size, and amylase and CEA negative.

Intraductal papillary mucinous neoplasms (IPMN) are epithelial pancreatic cystic tumors of mucin-producing cells that arise from the pancreatic ducts. They are most commonly seen in elderly patients, with sex distribution roughly balanced, a possible slight male predominance. IPMNs are slow growing tumors that have malignant potential and distinct variants have been described: main duct (IPMN 6 and 7), branch duct (IPMN 1, 3 and 4), and mixed branch and main duct (IPMN 2 and 5). Main duct IPMNs have a very high rate of malignancy (up to 70% in reported surgical series [8]); for this reason, the usual recommendation is surgical removal of the affected portion of the pancreas. Branch duct IPMNs are cystic neoplasms of the pancreas that have malignant potential and their management is challenging; the risk of surgery must be carefully weighed against the risk of malignancy when deciding on surgical removal or surveillance. This is the reason why great efforts are taken to distinguish mucinous cysts from other cyst lesions (specially, main duct IPMNs). All IPMNs are considered as premalignant cysts. They had the smallest size, between 2 and 3.5 cm. Four were amylase positive (above 250 U/L) and all were CEA positive (above 192 ng/mL or very closed in case of IPMN3 with 156 ng/mL).

Mucinous Cystadenoma (MCN) is another type of mucinous cystic neoplasm of the pancreas, traditionally considered typical of middle age females. MCN1 was 3 cm in size, amylase and CEA positive.

3.2. Analysis of TLB from Cystic Liquid Samples

TLB thermograms of 20 cystic fluid samples were obtained. Protein concentrations and dilutions could be considered, but in this case TLB curves were normalized according to their area under the curve values (AUC); therefore, signals from the different samples can be compared and uncertainties in protein concentration (inherent to colorimetric methods) are avoided. TLB cyst profiles clustered according to their clinical assessment (benign or premalignant nature) are represented in Figure 1.

Regarding the benign cystic group, the WOPN group exhibited a very similar cyst thermogram profile with two peaks at 65 and 82 °C. We can easily distinguish this group from the other benign cysts (Figure 2A). PC5 is the only PC lacking the 85 °C peak, and it is the only PC in a chronic pancreatitis context.

In the premalignant cyst group, branch duct IPMNs (IPMN1, IPMN3 and IPMN4) exhibited a similar profile (Figure 2C). Main duct IPMNs (IPMN6 and IPMN7) exhibited a single peak.

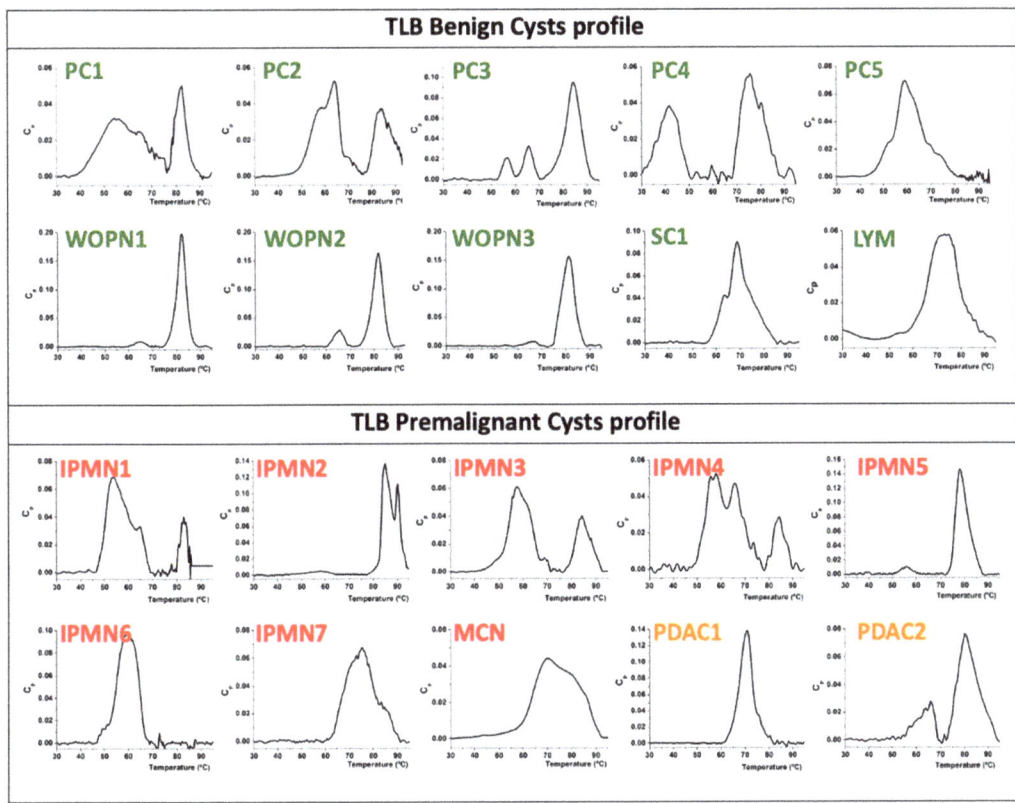

Figure 1. Individual TLB thermograms from cystic liquid samples. Samples were clustered according to their benign or premalignant nature.

3.3. Analysis of Proteomic Signatures from Cystic Liquid Samples

Proteins identified by LC-ESI-MS/MS (detailed in Table S1) were analyzed and clustered according to the benign or premalignant nature of the cyst (Figure 3). This first classification distinguishes 52 proteins common in the cyst groups, and 12 and 11 proteins present only in benign cysts and premalignant cysts, respectively. A deeper analysis according to different groups of cysts was performed.

3.3.1. Benign Cysts

The WOPN cyst group exhibited a homogeneous proteomic profile (Table S1). 18 out of 41 (44%) proteins were shared by all cysts in this group (Figure 4A). The similarity in these samples was even higher, because 10 more proteins were common in WOPN1 and WOPN3. Low protein concentration in WOPN2 (Figure S1A) could prevent proper identification of more proteins in that sample. The most abundant proteins found in this group were globulins (macroglobulin and immunoglobulins), a type of protein related to immunological response as a consequence of an inflammation process. This is consistent with the nature of this specific type of cyst: walled-off pancreatic necrosis (WOPN) is a well-circumscribed area of necrosis which occurs as a late complication of acute pancreatitis, generally after four weeks from the initial episode. Singular proteins detected in WOPN1 and WOPN3 samples were S-100 proteins. They belong to the S100 protein family, having important roles in inflammation and may also be useful markers for gut inflammation [37]. Once secreted in the extracellular space, S100A9 acts as a chemo-attractant, recruiting further inflammatory cells and creating an inflammatory microenvironment that promotes tumor development [38].

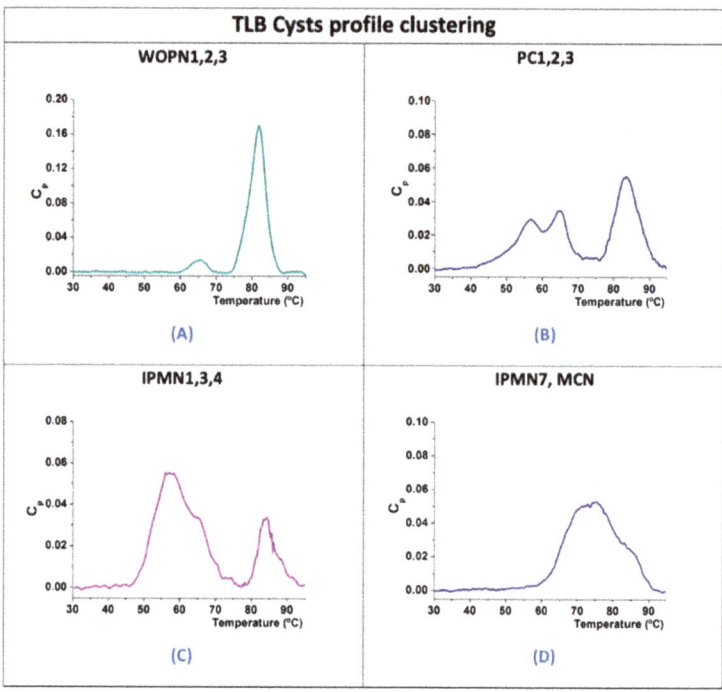

Figure 2. TLB thermograms from cystic liquid samples clustered according to their type. Average curves (colored lines) and standard deviations of curve values (grey) are represented: WOPNs (**A**), PCs (**B**), IPMNs (**C**) and IPMN7/MCNs (**D**).

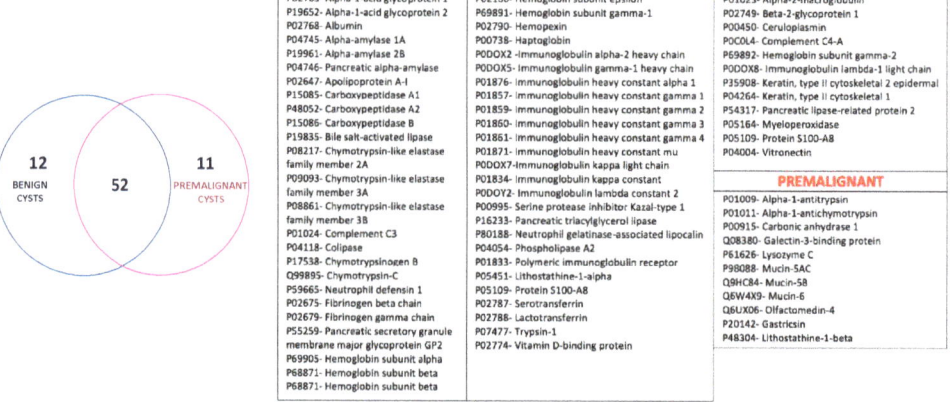

Figure 3. LC-ESI-MS/MS proteomic content of cystic samples. Common proteins were analyzed via Venn diagrams online tool (http://bioinformatics.psb.ugent.be/beg/tools/venn-diagrams). 12 and 11 proteins were detected only in benign cysts (blue) and premalignant cysts (pink), respectively, and 52 proteins appeared in both groups (intersection set). Table comprises the detailed information of the proteins in each set.

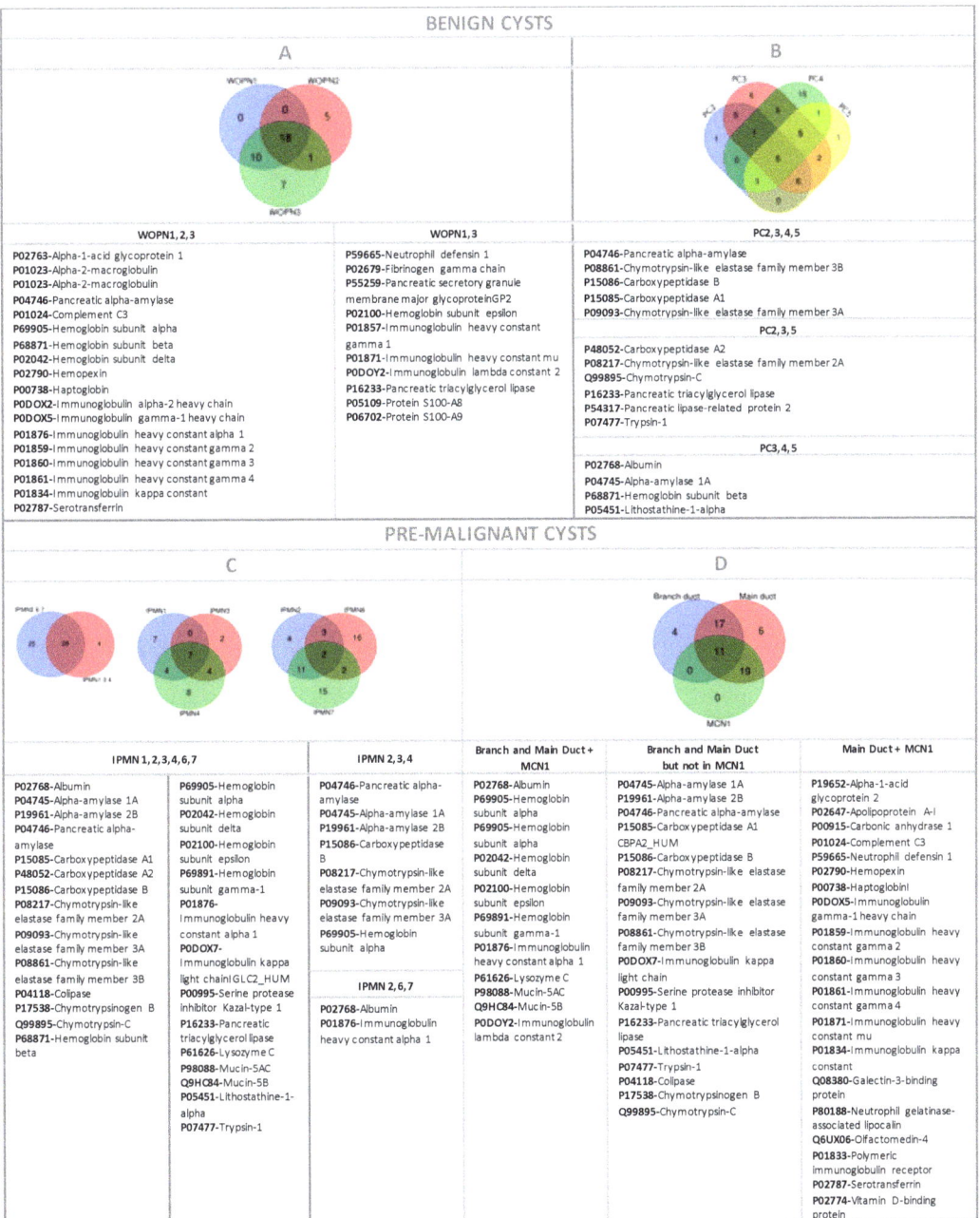

Figure 4. LC-ESI-MS/MS proteomic content of cystic samples according to cystic types: (**A**) WOPN, (**B**) PC, (**C**) IPMN, and (**D**) MCN+IPMN. Common proteins were analyzed via Venn diagrams online tool. Colors code for different groups and numbers inside each set and shared sub-sets indicate the number of identified proteins.

Common proteins of this group detected by electrophoresis (Figure S1A) are: proteolytic proteins, albumin, glycoside hydrolases, metalloproteases, immunoglobulins, and elastases. This agreed with the proteomic profile previously detailed (Table S1).

The homogeneity found in the proteomic signature of this group was reflected in the TLB cyst profiles of the cystic liquid (Figure 2A). As could be observed, compared to the rest of cystic groups studied in this work, these TLB cyst profiles represent a particular signature for WOPN cysts, easily distinguishing this group from the rest. They showed two peaks at $T_{1max} \approx 65\ °C$ and $T_{2max} \approx 81\ °C$, with a peak width at around $10\ °C$. Denatured proteins included in these peaks are detailed in Figure 4A.

In the PC cyst group, proteomic profiles data was also collected (Table S1), except for PC1, for which no protein was detected, except albumin. There are 5 proteins shared by all PCs (Figure 4B) and 10 proteins are shared by at least three PCs: PC2, PC3 and PC5 had 6 common proteins and PC3, PC4 and PC5 4 proteins. These cysts were negative for globulins (macroglobulin and immunoglobulins), indicating there were not any inflammatory processes going on (except for PC4, the rest of PCs in this subgroup were not in an acute pancreatitis context). The PC4 cyst, in acute pancreatitis context, exhibited 17 proteins not found in any other PCs (Table S1). It also contained a small number of carboxypeptidase or pancreatic elastase related proteins, absence of pancreatic triacylglycerol lipase and trypsin-1 and presence of globulins (macroglobulin and immunoglobulins), serotransferrin and lacto-transferrin, protein S100-A9, neutrophil defensin 1, and myeloperoxidase.

Common proteins of this group were detected in electrophoresis (Figure S1B) (except for PC1, where the total amount of protein was very low): glycoside hydrolases and metalloproteases (all PCs), proteolytic proteins (PC3 and PC4), albumin (all but PC2), lipases (all but PC5), immunoglobulins (PC3 and PC4) and elastases (PC2 and PC3). This was consistent with the proteomic profiles.

TLBs of PC cystic liquid (Figure 2B) were similar for PC1, PC2 and PC3, with three peaks at $T_{1max} \approx 55\ °C$, $T_{2max} \approx 65\ °C$ (two close peaks) and $T_{3max} \approx 85\ °C$ (peak width around $10\ °C$). Common proteins were found in these samples: amylase, IgGA, carboxypeptidase pancreatic elastase, chymo-trypsinogen, trypsin, glycoprotein GP2 and phospholipase A2. In PC5, $T_{3max} \approx 85\ °C$ was missing, and this could be the result of the absence of any of these proteins: IgGA, glycoprotein GP2, phospholipase A2 and chymo-trypsinogen. In PC4 there was a shift in the transitions, from 55 to $40\ °C$ and from 85 to $75\ °C$ (peak width was maintained in both cases).

In this group the clinical explanation for these differences could lie in the pancreatitis context for samples PC4 (acute) or PC5 (chronic).

3.3.2. Premalignant Cysts

The IPMN cyst group was more homogeneous from the clinical point of view. IPMN was the cystic group in this study with a number of proteins identified in the proteomic profile (Table S1). For example, it was not possible to identify proteins for IPMN5. One interesting observation was that none of the IPMNs contained globulins (macroglobulin or immunoglobulins), or they were negligible in other cyst groups, and only IPMN7 clearly contained them. These proteins are related to immunological responses as a consequence of inflammation and, therefore, it seemed that inflammation was not associated with this type of cyst.

Branch duct IPMNs (IPMN1, IPMN3 and IPMN4) shared 28 proteins with main duct IPMNs (IPMN2, IPMN6 and IPMN7) (Figure 4C). Branch duct IPMNs shared seven common proteins, and main duct IPMNs shared only two proteins. Neither of these proteins were unique in any of the two groups (they were included in the 28 proteins in common).

Common proteins of this group detected in the electrophoresis gel are albumin and immunoglobulins (IPMN1, IPMN2 and IPMN5); glycoside hydrolases and elastases (IPMN1, IPMN3, IPMN4 and IPMN5); metalloproteases (IPMN1 and IPMN3); and lipases (IPMN3 and IPMN4). Proteolytic proteins were not present in any of IPMNs samples (Figure S1D). This was consistent with the proteomic profiles.

TLBs of IPMN cystic liquid (Figure 2C) were similar for IPMN1, IPMN3 and IPMN4, all being branch duct IPMNs. They exhibited two close peaks (around $T_{1max} \approx 55\ °C$, $T_{2max} \approx 65\ °C$) and a third peak at $T_{3max} \approx 85\ °C$ (peak width around $10\ °C$). These peaks could correspond to the common proteins found in this group (amylases, carboxypeptidase and pancreatic elastases).

TLB of main duct type IPMN cystic liquids had a wider single peak at $\approx 55\ °C$ and $\approx 75\ °C$ for IPMN6 or IPMN7, respectively.

TLB of mixed type IPMN cystic liquids presented characteristics from both branch or duct IPMN groups with a low signal peak at $\approx 55\ °C$ and one peak at $\approx 80\ °C$ for IPMN5, or two peaks at $\approx 85\ °C$ and $90\ °C$ for IPMN2.

There was no proteomic profile available for IPMN5, but, according to electrophoresis, there was no protein from the amylase family, and additionally IPMN 2 and IPMN 7 lacked amylases, carboxy-peptidase and pancreatic elastases. These three cysts did not exhibit any peak (or it was neglectable) at $\approx 55\ °C$.

The MCN 1 cyst was in the mixed cysts group, but it had a premalignant nature.

MCN1 shared 11 proteins with IPMNs, either branch or main duct type, (Figure 4D) and 19 more proteins in common only with main duct IPMNs (Figure 4D) with five of these protein shared with IPMN7. When comparing MCN1 and IPMN7 profiles (Table S1), 15 common proteins were found. In fact, IPMN7 was the only IPMN cyst showing globulins (macroglobulin and immunoglobulins). In addition, protein profile in electrophoresis for MCN1 was similar to IPMNs (Figure S1E). However, 17 proteins were detected in IPMNs, but not in MCN1. There were no proteins shared only with branch duct IPMNs.

When comparing MCN1 and IPMN7 profiles (Table S1), 15 common proteins were found. In fact, IPMN7 was the only IPMN cyst showing globulins (macroglobulin and immunoglobulins).

Proteins detected in electrophoresis for MCN1 were similar to IPMNs (Figure S1E).

TLB for cystic liquid sample exhibited a wide transition (around $30\ °C$ width) with two peaks (around $T_{1max} \approx 70\ °C$, $T_{2max} \approx 85\ °C$), very similar to the IPMN7 profile (Figure 2D). MCN1 did not exhibit any peak at around $55\ °C$ and, again, no amylases, carboxypeptidase or pancreatic elastases were detected by proteomics.

Mixed Cyst Group was a completely heterogenous group comprising a serous cyst, a lymphocele, and two samples of pancreatic ductal adenocarcinoma (PDCA) (which cannot be considered as a cyst).

SC and LYM: The main difference between serous cyst and lymphocele (cystic benign samples), compared to the rest of samples, was the presence of apolipoprotein A-I (only MCN1 and IPMN7 seemed to contain it) (Table S1). In addition, they were positive for globulins (macroglobulin and immunoglobulins), as with the samples with an active inflammatory process. Some typical pancreatic cystic proteins were missing: amylase, metalloproteases, lipases, elastases. Some of these proteins were already employed as clinical biomarkers for pancreatic cyst diagnosis [9], such as amylase.

Common proteins of this group detected in electrophoresis are: serotransferrin, albumin, lipoproteins and immunoglobulins (Figure S1C). This agreed with the proteomic profiles.

All TLB cyst profiles in this group showed particular features and looked different from the other cystic profiles. They exhibited one single peak: SC at $T_{1max} \approx 70\ °C$ (peak width around $20\ °C$) and LYM at $T_{1max} \approx 75\ °C$ (peak width around $25\ °C$). Common proteins (Table S1) are albumin, lipoproteins, hemoglobins, globulins, and serotransferrin.

PDACs: Proteomic profiles of PDACs (Figure S2) showed 20 shared proteins from hemoglobin, immune-globulins and transferrin groups. PDAC1 also contained other proteins, and PDAC2 contained proteins we previously identified in cysts, such as amylases, metalloproteases, lipases, elastases.

TLB cyst profile in PDAC1 exhibited one peak ($T_{1max} \approx 70\ °C$) and PDAC2 showed two peaks ($T_{1max} \approx 65\ °C$ and $T_{2max} \approx 80\ °C$) (Figure 1). This difference could be related to the different proteomic profile between the two samples mentioned above. Electrophoresis also confirmed this different pattern (Figure S1F).

3.4. Analysis of TLB from Serum Samples

TLB thermograms from serum samples were obtained. The goal was to search for any potential reflection of the cystic pathology in plasmatic serum. TLB serum profiles were normalized according to their area under the curve values (AUC), again avoiding protein concentration influence. Then, they were clustered according to the clinical assessment of the cyst (Figure 5). We focused our attention on distinguishing between premalignant and benign cysts. Unfortunately, it was not possible to obtain serum samples at the same time as the eco-endoscopy procedure for all the patients included in this study.

PCs are benign lesions found in the context of acute or chronic pancreatitis. It has been previously reported that inflammatory processes can be reflected in TLB serum profile [23]. According to the PC TLB serum thermograms, they seemed to be somewhat different (Figure 5A).

IPMNs, being premalignant lesions, could also exhibit some distinctive features compared to healthy patients in their TLB serum profile on the basis of the previous studies on TLB applied to cancer diagnosis [30,33,34]. Apparently, in the case of IPMNs, TLB serum profiles, except for IPMN7, seem quite similar to healthy controls (Figure 5B).

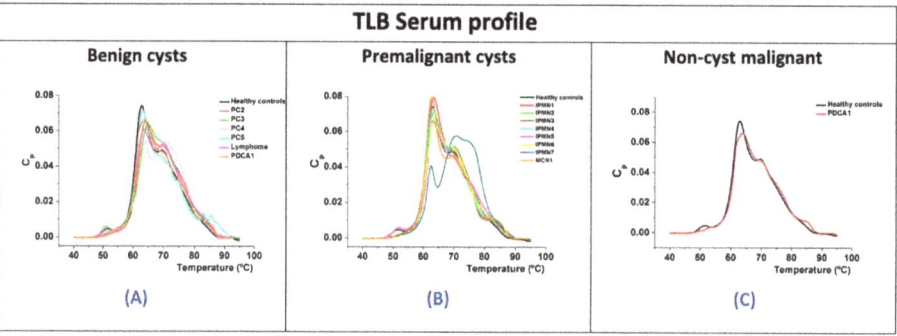

Figure 5. Examples of serum TLB thermograms from different types of cystic patients, clustered according to cyst types: premalignant (**A**), benign (**B**) and non-cyst malignant (**C**). Typical TLB thermogram for a healthy subject is represented with black line in (**A–C**).

The multiparametric analysis previously developed in our group [30] was applied to TLB serum profiles. The purpose was to help in the identification of cystic disease-related TLB features and the quantification of the TLB serum score for patients' serum (Table S2). Mono-variant analysis of the individual TLB parameters obtained from the thermograms showed that 6 out of 15 parameters were statistically different (p-value < 0.05). Only these six parameters were used to construct the classification model and calculate the TLB serum score for each sample, as previously described in [33].

According to the results in Figure 6, the TLB serum score comparison between healthy subjects and cyst patients (both, benign and premalignant) indicated that the differences were statistically significant using the Wilcoxon test (p-value < 0.001). Similarly, TLB serum score could differentiate between healthy subjects and benign cyst patients (p-value < 0.001), and between healthy subjects and premalignant cyst patients (p-value < 0.001).

TLB serum score values are between 0 and 1: the closer to 0, the smaller the alterations in plasma (healthy status), while the closer to 1, the larger the alterations in plasma (diseased status). TLB serum score values were mainly under 0.5 for healthy (82 out of 84, 98% true negative rate) and over 0.5 for cysts patients (10 out 14, 71% true positive rate). This meant that this score may be useful for detecting the presence of cystic lesion. The area under the ROC curve is 0.94 (Figure S3) with sensitivity of 71%, specificity of 98%, a positive predictive value (PPV) of 83%, and a negative predictive value (NPV) of 98%. Unfortunately, there was no statistical difference between both cysts' groups; that is, TLB serum score did not discriminate between benign and premalignant cysts (p-value = 0.501).

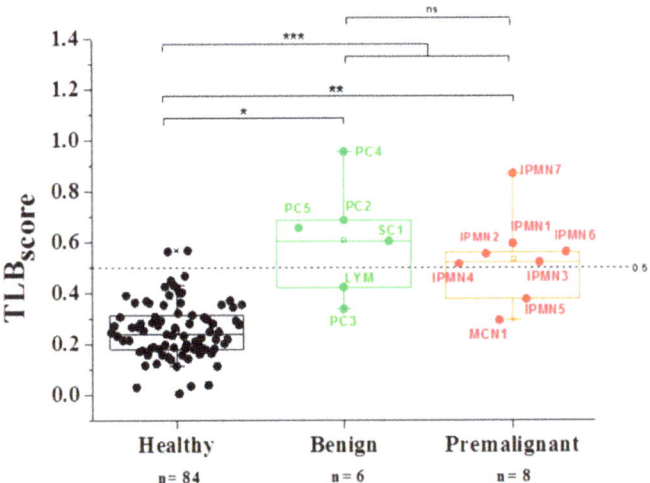

Figure 6. TLB serum score from serum TLB profiles from healthy controls and both types of cysts (benign and premalignant). Median values were compared using the Wilcoxon test: * p-value$_{healthy-benign}$ = 0.00026; ** p-value$_{healthy-premalignant}$ = 0.000057; *** p-value$_{healthy-cysts}$ = 0.0000012; ns p-value$_{benign-premalignant}$ = 0.501.

TLB serum values closest to 1 in PC corresponded to those associated to the acute or chronic pancreatitis context (inflammatory process can be reflected in serum).

TLB serum values of IPMN were around 0.5 (except in IPMN7). CEA value for IPMN7 was over 50,000 ng/mL, the highest of all premalignant cysts.

All types of cyst could be clustered differentially from healthy controls by using this single TLB serum score. These results agreed with our previously published results on lung cancer disease [33] in which TLB serum score was able to discriminate between diseased and healthy subjects.

Cystic pathologies are local lesions for which a systemic reflection in blood might not be expected. However, if cystic pathology is accompanied by inflammation, blood alterations may be important, even for a benign lesion.

As a further development, in this study we also proposed to evaluate whether TLB serum score could provide useful information to gastroenterologists for the diagnosis before and besides endoscopic ultrasound procedures. Despite the small number of samples (14 serum samples from cyst patients), a restricted TLB serum score excluding healthy control subjects and considering benign cysts as control samples was performed. Benign and premalignant cysts were 43% and 57% of the samples, respectively. First, we performed a mono-variant analysis of TLB parameters (Table S3) and none of the individual parameters was statistically different (p-values > 0.05). Therefore, only parameters presenting p-value below 0.25 were considered in constructing the classification model and calculating this new TLB serum score (benign vs. premalignant cysts). For a TLB score threshold of 0.5, 4 out 6 (67%) benign cysts had a TLB score below 0.5, and 6 out 8 (75%) premalignant cysts had a TLB score above 0.5. The area under the ROC curve is 0.875 (Figure 7B) with sensitivity of 75%, specificity of 67%, a positive predictive value (PPV) of 75% and a negative predictive value (NPV) of 67%. When using the Youden index as a threshold (0.75), all benign samples were well classified (TLB score below 0.75).

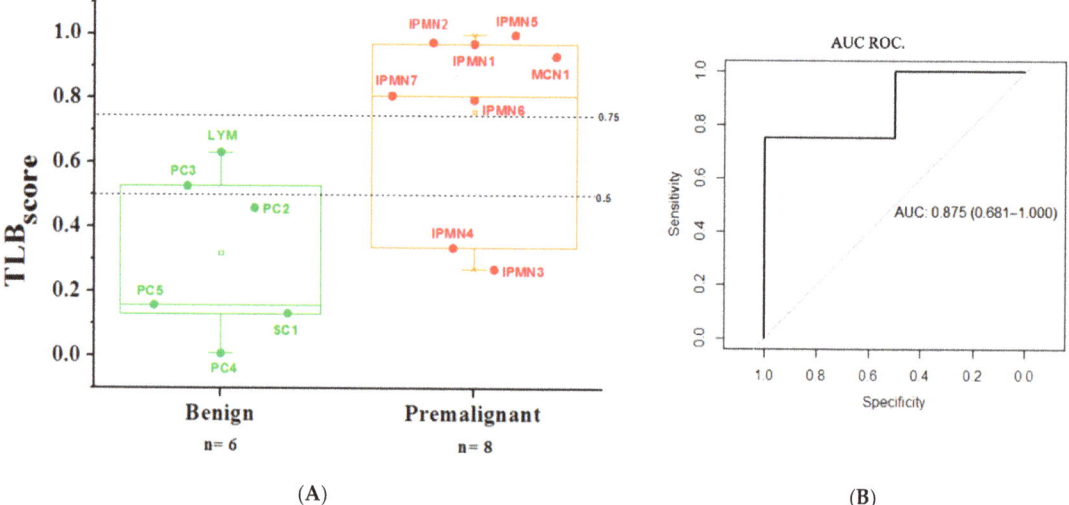

Figure 7. (**A**)/TLB serum score parameters from serum TLB serum profiles from benign and premalignant cyst patients. (**B**)/ROC curve illustrating the statistical performance of TLB serum score (benign vs. premalignant cysts). AUC = Area Under Curve (95%CI).

4. Discussion

Pancreatic neoplasms are generally discovered incidentally and consists of IPMNs, predominantly [7]. The diagnosis of malignant IPMN lesions involves a certain degree of subjectivity and variability, which is undesirable for clinical practice, due to the lack of standardized guidelines. Thus, there is a necessity of new diagnosis tools to differentiate between benign and premalignant pancreatic cysts to help in making decisions about surgical intervention or periodic surveillance.

The analysis of cyst fluid may provide information regarding established biomarkers that helps the physician in the diagnosis [13,39]. This type of biological sample includes a diverse amount and type of proteins, representing an interesting challenge for thermal liquid biopsy. TLB for blood serum samples has been proven useful for different types of cancer, and premalignant pancreatic cysts will eventually evolve to pancreatic cancer. Additionally, TLB has been applied to other body fluids (serum, plasma, urine, synovial and cerebrospinal fluids [25,31,40,41], or even tumor digestion), provided that the TLB thermogram is a reflection of the protein composition, interactions, and modifications in the complex sample [32]. Similarities in protein composition of cysts (which is a known biomarker for cyst classification) will result in similarities in TLB cyst profiles, thus, providing the basis for a diagnostic procedure based on TLB. As has been previously described, TLB cyst profile reflects protein composition, but also protein interactions. The presence or absence of a certain protein could promote changes in the profile for other proteins in the sample, especially if they were interacting (interactome concept) [25]. Similar effects could be envisaged for protein modifications as a result of metabolic or pathologic processes.

In our study, we recruited 20 patients who, after being diagnosed with a cystic lesion by CT scan or MNR, underwent routine endoscopic ultrasonography where a sample of cyst fluid was obtained. The final clinical diagnosis of the lesions found was based on the different clinical features of the patient (fluid aspect, biochemical biomarkers and pathological anatomy results) according to current clinical guidelines [8,36].

To our knowledge, this was the first time that pancreatic cyst fluid was characterized using a TLB technique and thermal profiles were clustered according to the clinical information on the cysts. We confirmed that cyst liquid thermograms reflect protein content in the samples. There was a high intra-group variability within the TLB cyst thermograms. Only WOPN cysts could be easily differentiated from PCs, because there was a clear profile type that could be associated with them (Figure 2A) and they also shared 18 proteins (Figure 4A). More samples are required to clearly define a common cyst thermogram for benign or premalignant cysts. Having the TLB thermogram available for specialist appraisal, perhaps the diagnosis could be oriented to the MCN cyst type. As we have already discussed, there is a considerable subjective component in the physician diagnosis, and the more complementary tools available for a better discrimination, the better for the gastroenterologist in producing an appropriate evaluation statement.

Another goal of this study was linking cyst thermograms to proteomic signatures of cyst samples, bearing in mind that, as we said before, TLB cyst profile reflects sample composition and also potential interactions and modifications in proteins. Each protein unfolds in a certain manner and the calorimetric cyst profile obtained is characteristic for that unfolding process. When two or more proteins are together in the same sample, the resulting profile will be the sum of the signal of the independent profiles when proteins are not interacting; or, in case the proteins interact, the resulting profile could change [42].

A deeper analysis of the proteomic profile of pancreatic intra-cyst sample can be found in the literature [43]. We used proteomic identification to assess the correlation between the TLB thermograms and the protein content. The TLB methodology is based on apparently simple curves, but they contain relevant information for diagnosis.

This is clear when looking at WOPN samples (as we already described above): TLB thermograms were quite similar and overlapped, and proteomic profiles also confirmed this similarity. Nevertheless, results are not so clear for the rest of the cyst groups and further studies to increase the number of intra-cyst samples are needed.

This pilot study reveals some interesting aspects. In IPMN, less inflammatory process indicators have been detected, specifically less immunoglobulins in comparison to benign cysts. There were also less proteins related to iron metabolism (serotransferrin, lactotransferrin, ferritin, hemopexin and haptoglobin) which has been referenced as an indicator of health alteration [44,45].

The information obtained through the cyst TLB thermogram is not focused on the detection of a specific biomarker but comprises information about a large amount of proteins and their relations (interactions and modifications), which could be interesting when doubts about the diagnosis of a cyst are cast. This study represents a proof of concept to confirm that TLB cyst thermograms contain valuable information. According to these preliminary results, a further, larger study can lead to the establishment of certain specific profiles for different type of cysts and can help during diagnosis.

The analysis of a cyst fluid sample implies that the patient has undergone an endoscopic ultrasonography procedure, a risky, invasive test that nowadays is the only way to achieve a reasonably accurate diagnosis of the benign or premalignant nature of cysts. Here we wondered if alterations due to the cyst could have a systemic reflection in blood serum, and whether or not they could be detected through TLB. If metabolic alterations in cyst fluid are translated into blood serum alterations, a quick, low-risk, minimally invasive tool to obtain information on the cyst would be available to differentiate between healthy/cystic patients and/or benign/premalignant cystic patients. TLB has been previously applied in our lab to study different type of tumor disease such as gastric, lung cancer or melanoma [30,33,34]. In the present study, we also obtained 15 serum samples from the 20 patients and their TLB serum profiles were obtained (Figure 5). As normally occurs with TLB serum thermograms, it is difficult to visually discriminate and distinguish among patients' profiles. In previous studies from our group, we contributed to develop, first, a multiparametric analysis [30] and, later, a TLB serum score [33] to manage and assess TLB thermograms according to a simple interpretation index (TLB serum score from 0 to 1) that could be implemented in diagnosis, easily allowing the stratification of the patients.

We first compared the TLB serum thermograms from patients to thermograms from healthy subjects that were not suffering from the disease. We applied a general TLB serum score previously reported [33] and the results were statistically different when comparing healthy subjects with benign or malignant cyst patients, individually or together as a pooled group of patients (p-values lower than 0.05) (Figure 6). Specificity and sensitivity values (98% and 71%, respectively), as well as PPV and NPV values (83% and 98%, respectively), were quite high.

TLB serum scores (from benign or premalignant cyst groups) were not statistically different when using the TLB general formula when comparing to healthy subjects. Therefore, on that basis it was not possible to distinguish between both types of cyst. Therefore, we focused our attention on specifically comparing both patients' groups and obtaining a cyst-specific TLB serum score that could be applied to evaluate intra-group cyst patient variability. This new TLB serum score would strengthen the discrimination power, based on the specific parameters reflecting differences between cysts. The challenge is considerable, because a mono-variant analysis of cyst TLB parameters (Table S3) showed that none of the individual parameters was statistically different between the benign and premalignant cyst group. As we previously confirmed in our studies, the combination of all the parameters in a multiparametric-based single TLB serum score increased the discrimination ability. Despite the small patient sample cohort, it was possible to distinguish between benign and premalignant cysts. This specific TLB serum score (values from 0 to 1) were over 0.75 (according to Youden) in 6 out of 8 (75%) premalignant samples, while TLB serum scores were below 0.75 in 6 out of 6 (100%) benign samples. The diagnosis accuracy based in the area under the curve (AUC) was 0.875, a promising starting point for extending the study. Therefore, more serum samples from patients with pancreatic cysts should be included in a larger future study, but these preliminary results are promising and allow us to foresee that the TLB serum score could be applied routinely in the clinic as an additional complementary tool helping physicians in making better diagnostic decisions.

5. Conclusions

TLB analysis can be applied to both plasmatic serum and cyst fluid as a sort of high information content tool. Despite the small number of samples in this pilot study, it represents a proof of concept for developing a useful technique for classifying and evaluating risk in pancreatic cysts based on liquid biopsy in both body fluids. A future, larger study, with a larger number of samples for each cyst category, could confirm whether TLB of plasma or cyst fluid could be a new diagnosis tool to differentiate between benign and premalignant pancreatic cysts to help clinician gastroenterologists in making decisions about disease management. In case of serum, TLB would represent a quick, low-risk, minimally invasive tool easily translated to clinical practice for diagnosis and patient monitoring. In addition, TLB is reasonably cheap for serum tests (an estimated cost of 100–200 €/$ per test, although with a higher cost for cyst fluid test), and could be performed with predefined frequency for patient surveillance.

Supplementary Materials: The following are available online at https://www.mdpi.com/2075-4426/11/1/25/s1, Figure S1: Electrophoresis analysis of proteomic profiles, Figure S2: LC-ESI-MS/MS proteomic content of cyst samples types identification, Figure S3: ROC curve illustrating the statistical performance of TLB serum score (healthy vs. cysts); Table S1: Detailed information of cyst proteomic profiles, Table S2: Mono-variant analysis of TLB parameters of healthy controls and cysts patients, Table S3: Mono-variant analysis of TLB parameters of benign and premalignant cysts patients.

Author Contributions: Conceptualization, A.V.-C., and O.A.; methodology, S.H.-D., J.L.O., O.S.-G., A.V.-C., and O.A.; software, S.H.-D., J.L.O., O.S.-G., A.V.-C., and O.A.; validation, J.L.O., S.V., O.S.-G., A.V.-C., and O.A.; formal analysis, J.L.O., S.V., O.S.-G., O.A., and A.V.-C.; investigation, L.C, S.V., A.V.-C., and O.A.; resources, G.G.-R., J.L.O., O.S.-G., Á.L., C.S., A.V.-C., and O.A.; data curation, S.H.-D., G.G.-R., C.S., J.L.O., and O.A.; writing—original draft preparation, S.H.-D., L.C.-L., J.L.O., A.V.-C., and O.A.; writing—review and editing, S.H.-D., G.G.-R., L.C.-L., J.L.O., S.V., O.S.-G., Á.L., J.M., A.V.-C., and O.A.; visualization, J.L.O., L.C.-L., O.S.-G., A.V.-C., and O.A.; supervision, Á.L., A.V.-C., and O.A.; project administration, O.A. and A.V.-C.; funding acquisition, Á.L., O.A., and A.V.-C. All authors have read and agreed to the published version of the manuscript.

Funding: This research was funded by the Spanish Ministry of Economy and Competitiveness and European ERDF Funds (MCIU/AEI/FEDER, EU) (BFU2016-78232-P to A.V.C.); Projects funded by Instituto de Salud Carlos III and co-funded by European Union (ESF, "Investing in your future"): "PI15/00663 (FIS project to O.A)", "PI18/00349 (FIS project to O.A. and Contract to LC)", "FI19/00146 (PFIS contract for SHD)", "CPII13/00017 (Miguel Servet Program to OA)"; Diputación General de Aragón (Protein Targets and Bioactive Compounds Group E45_17R to A.V.C. and Digestive Pathology Group B25_17R to O.A.); and the Centro de Investigación Biomédica en Red en Enfermedades Hepáticas y Digestivas (CIBERehd).

Institutional Review Board Statement: The study was conducted in accordance with the Declaration of Helsinki, and the protocol was approved by the Ethics Committee of CEICA (PI16/0228).

Informed Consent Statement: All subjects gave their informed consent for inclusion before they participated in the study.

Data Availability Statement: The data presented in this study are available on request from the corresponding author.

Acknowledgments: Proteomic analyses were performed in the Proteomics Platform of Servicios Científico Técnicos del CIBA (IACS-Universidad de Zaragoza), ProteoRed ISCIII member, Zaragoza, Spain.

Conflicts of Interest: The authors declare no conflict of interest.

References

1. De Jong, K.; Nio, C.Y.; Hermans, J.J.; Dijkgraaf, M.G.; Gouma, D.J.; van Eijck, C.H.; van Heel, E.; Klass, G.; Fockens, P.; Bruno, M.J. High prevalence of pancreatic cysts detected by screening magnetic resonance imaging examinations. *Clin. Gastroenterol. Hepatol.* **2010**, *8*, 806–811. [CrossRef] [PubMed]
2. Megibow, A.J.; Baker, M.E.; Gore, R.M.; Taylor, A. The incidental pancreatic cyst. *Radiol. Clin. N. Am.* **2011**, *49*, 349–359. [CrossRef] [PubMed]
3. Klibansky, D.A.; Reid-Lombardo, K.M.; Gordon, S.R.; Gardner, T.B. The clinical relevance of the increasing incidence of intraductal papillary mucinous neoplasm. *Clin. Gastroenterol. Hepatol.* **2012**, *10*, 555–558. [CrossRef] [PubMed]
4. Jacobson, B.C.; Baron, T.H.; Adler, D.G.; Davila, R.E.; Egan, J.; Hirota, W.K.; Leighton, J.A.; Qureshi, W.; Rajan, E.; Zuckerman, M.J.; et al. ASGE guideline: The role of endoscopy in the diagnosis and the management of cystic lesions and inflammatory fluid collections of the pancreas. *Gastrointest. Endosc.* **2005**, *61*, 363–370. [CrossRef]
5. Tanaka, M.; Chari, S.; Adsay, V.; Fernandez-del Castillo, C.; Falconi, M.; Shimizu, M.; Yamaguchi, K.; Yamao, K.; Matsuno, S. International consensus guidelines for management of intraductal papillary mucinous neoplasms and mucinous cystic neoplasms of the pancreas. *Pancreatology* **2006**, *6*, 17–32. [CrossRef]
6. Khalid, A.; Brugge, W. ACG practice guidelines for the diagnosis and management of neoplastic pancreatic cysts. *Am. J. Gastroenterol.* **2007**, *102*, 2339–2349. [CrossRef]
7. Tanaka, M.; Fernandez-del Castillo, C.; Adsay, V.; Chari, S.; Falconi, M.; Jang, J.Y.; Kimura, W.; Levy, P.; Pitman, M.B.; Schmidt, C.M.; et al. International consensus guidelines 2012 for the management of IPMN and MCN of the pancreas. *Pancreatology* **2012**, *12*, 183–197. [CrossRef]
8. Tanaka, M.; Fernández-Del Castillo, C.; Kamisawa, T.; Jang, J.Y.; Levy, P.; Ohtsuka, T.; Salvia, R.; Shimizu, Y.; Tada, M.; Wolfgang, C.L. Revisions of international consensus Fukuoka guidelines for the management of IPMN of the pancreas. In *Pancreatology*, © *2017 IAP and EPC*; Elsevier: Amsterdam, The Netherlands, 2017; Volume 17, pp. 738–753.
9. European evidence-based guidelines on pancreatic cystic neoplasms. *Gut* **2018**, *67*, 789–804. [CrossRef]
10. Brugge, W.R.; Lauwers, G.Y.; Sahani, D.; Fernandez-del Castillo, C.; Warshaw, A.L. Cystic neoplasms of the pancreas. *N. Engl. J. Med.* **2004**, *351*, 1218–1226. [CrossRef]
11. Muthusamy, V.R.; Chandrasekhara, V.; Acosta, R.D.; Bruining, D.H.; Chathadi, K.V.; Eloubeidi, M.A.; Faulx, A.L.; Fonkalsrud, L.; Gurudu, S.R.; Khashab, M.A.; et al. The role of endoscopy in the diagnosis and treatment of cystic pancreatic neoplasms. *Gastrointest. Endosc.* **2016**, *84*, 1–9. [CrossRef]

12. Van der Waaij, L.A.; van Dullemen, H.M.; Porte, R.J. Cyst fluid analysis in the differential diagnosis of pancreatic cystic lesions: A pooled analysis. *Gastrointest. Endosc.* **2005**, *62*, 383–389. [CrossRef]
13. Rogart, J.N.; Loren, D.E.; Singu, B.S.; Kowalski, T.E. Cyst wall puncture and aspiration during EUS-guided fine needle aspiration may increase the diagnostic yield of mucinous cysts of the pancreas. *J. Clin. Gastroenterol.* **2011**, *45*, 164–169. [CrossRef] [PubMed]
14. Jang, J.W.; Kim, M.H.; Jeong, S.U.; Kim, J.; Park, D.H.; Lee, S.S.; Seo, D.W.; Lee, S.K.; Kim, J.H. Clinical characteristics of intraductal papillary mucinous neoplasm manifesting as acute pancreatitis or acute recurrent pancreatitis. *J. Gastroenterol. Hepatol.* **2013**, *28*, 731–738. [CrossRef]
15. Brugge, W.R.; Lewandrowski, K.; Lee-Lewandrowski, E.; Centeno, B.A.; Szydlo, T.; Regan, S.; del Castillo, C.F.; Warshaw, A.L. Diagnosis of pancreatic cystic neoplasms: A report of the cooperative pancreatic cyst study. *Gastroenterology* **2004**, *126*, 1330–1336. [CrossRef] [PubMed]
16. Singh, H.; McGrath, K.; Singhi, A.D. Novel Biomarkers for Pancreatic Cysts. *Dig. Dis. Sci.* **2017**, *62*, 1796–1807. [CrossRef]
17. Kaplan, J.H.; Gonda, T.A. The Use of Biomarkers in the Risk Stratification of Cystic Neoplasms. *Gastrointest. Endosc. Clin. N. Am.* **2018**, *28*, 549–568. [CrossRef]
18. Moris, D.; Damaskos, C.; Spartalis, E.; Papalampros, A.; Vernadakis, S.; Dimitroulis, D.; Griniatsos, J.; Felekouras, E.; Nikiteas, N. Updates and Critical Evaluation on Novel Biomarkers for the Malignant Progression of Intraductal Papillary Mucinous Neoplasms of the Pancreas. *Anticancer Res.* **2017**, *37*, 2185–2194. [CrossRef]
19. Soyer, O.M.; Baran, B.; Ormeci, A.C.; Sahin, D.; Gokturk, S.; Evirgen, S.; Basar, R.; Firat, P.; Akyuz, F.; Demir, K.; et al. Role of biochemistry and cytological analysis of cyst fluid for the differential diagnosis of pancreatic cysts: A retrospective cohort study. *Medicine* **2017**, *96*, e5513. [CrossRef]
20. Levy, A.; Popovici, T.; Bories, P.N. Tumor markers in pancreatic cystic fluids for diagnosis of malignant cysts. *Int. J. Biol. Markers* **2017**, *32*, e291–e296. [CrossRef]
21. Ngamruengphong, S.; Lennon, A.M. Analysis of Pancreatic Cyst Fluid. *Surg. Pathol. Clin.* **2016**, *9*, 677–684. [CrossRef]
22. Garbett, N.C.; Miller, J.J.; Jenson, A.B.; Chaires, J.B. Calorimetric analysis of the plasma proteome. *Semin. Nephrol.* **2007**, *27*, 621–626. [CrossRef] [PubMed]
23. Garbett, N.C.; Miller, J.J.; Jenson, A.B.; Chaires, J.B. Calorimetry outside the box: A new window into the plasma proteome. *Biophys. J.* **2008**, *94*, 1377–1383. [CrossRef] [PubMed]
24. Garbett, N.C.; Mekmaysy, C.S.; Helm, C.W.; Jenson, A.B.; Chaires, J.B. Differential scanning calorimetry of blood plasma for clinical diagnosis and monitoring. *Exp. Mol. Pathol.* **2009**, *86*, 186–191. [CrossRef] [PubMed]
25. Garbett, N.C.; Merchant, M.L.; Helm, C.W.; Jenson, A.B.; Klein, J.B.; Chaires, J.B. Detection of cervical cancer biomarker patterns in blood plasma and urine by differential scanning calorimetry and mass spectrometry. *PLoS ONE* **2014**, *9*, e84710. [CrossRef]
26. Garbett, N.C.; Brock, G.N. Differential scanning calorimetry as a complementary diagnostic tool for the evaluation of biological samples. *Biochim. Biophys. Acta* **2016**, *1860*, 981–989. [CrossRef]
27. Todinova, S.; Krumova, S.; Kurtev, P.; Dimitrov, V.; Djongov, L.; Dudunkov, Z.; Taneva, S.G. Calorimetry-based profiling of blood plasma from colorectal cancer patients. *Biochim. Biophys. Acta* **2012**, *1820*, 1879–1885. [CrossRef]
28. Todinova, S.; Krumova, S.; Radoeva, R.; Gartcheva, L.; Taneva, S.G. Calorimetric markers of Bence Jones and nonsecretory multiple myeloma serum proteome. *Anal. Chem.* **2014**, *86*, 12355–12361. [CrossRef]
29. Todinova, S.; Krumova, S.; Danailova, A.; Petkova, V.; Guenova, M.; Mihaylov, G.; Gartcheva, L.; Taneva, S.G. Calorimetric markers for monitoring of multiple myeloma and Waldenstrom's macroglobulinemia patients. *Eur. Biophys. J.* **2018**, *47*, 549–559. [CrossRef]
30. Vega, S.; Garcia-Gonzalez, M.A.; Lanas, A.; Velazquez-Campoy, A.; Abian, O. Deconvolution analysis for classifying gastric adenocarcinoma patients based on differential scanning calorimetry serum thermograms. *Sci. Rep.* **2015**, *5*, 7988. [CrossRef]
31. Chagovetz, A.A.; Jensen, R.L.; Recht, L.; Glantz, M.; Chagovetz, A.M. Preliminary use of differential scanning calorimetry of cerebrospinal fluid for the diagnosis of glioblastoma multiforme. *J. Neurooncol.* **2011**, *105*, 499–506. [CrossRef]
32. Chagovetz, A.A.; Quinn, C.; Damarse, N.; Hansen, L.D.; Chagovetz, A.M.; Jensen, R.L. Differential scanning calorimetry of gliomas: A new tool in brain cancer diagnostics? *Neurosurgery* **2013**, *73*, 289–295, discussion 295. [CrossRef] [PubMed]
33. Rodrigo, A.; Ojeda, J.L.; Vega, S.; Sanchez-Gracia, O.; Lanas, A.; Isla, D.; Velazquez-Campoy, A.; Abian, O. Thermal Liquid Biopsy (TLB): A Predictive Score Derived from Serum Thermograms as a Clinical Tool for Screening Lung Cancer Patients. *Cancers* **2019**, *11*, 12. [CrossRef] [PubMed]
34. Velazquez-Campoy, A.; Vega, S.; Sanchez-Gracia, O.; Lanas, A.; Rodrigo, A.; Kaliappan, A.; Hall, M.B.; Nguyen, T.Q.; Brock, G.N.; Chesney, J.A.; et al. Thermal liquid biopsy for monitoring melanoma patients under surveillance during treatment: A pilot study. *Biochim. Biophys. Acta Gen. Subj.* **2018**, *1862*, 1701–1710. [CrossRef] [PubMed]
35. Rodrigo, A.; Abian, O.; Velázquez-Campoy, A.; Callejo, A.; Vega-Sánchez, S.; Fernandez, A.; Sánchez-Gracia, O.; Iranzo, P.; Cruellas, M.; Quilez, E.; et al. Liquid thermal biopsy as a new non-invasive method of diagnosis for lung cancer patients. *J. Clin. Oncol.* **2018**, *36*, e21207. [CrossRef]
36. Banks, P.A.; Bollen, T.L.; Dervenis, C.; Gooszen, H.G.; Johnson, C.D.; Sarr, M.G.; Tsiotos, G.G.; Vege, S.S.; Group, A.P.C.W. Classification of acute pancreatitis—2012: Revision of the Atlanta classification and definitions by international consensus. *Gut* **2013**, *62*, 102–111. [CrossRef]
37. Leach, S.T.; Day, A.S. S100 proteins in the pathogenesis and diagnosis of inflammatory bowel disease. *Expert Rev. Clin. Immunol.* **2006**, *2*, 471–480. [CrossRef]

38. Nedjadi, T.; Evans, A.; Sheikh, A.; Barerra, L.; Al-Ghamdi, S.; Oldfield, L.; Greenhalf, W.; Neoptolemos, J.P.; Costello, E. S100A8 and S100A9 proteins form part of a paracrine feedback loop between pancreatic cancer cells and monocytes. *BMC Cancer* **2018**, *18*, 1255. [CrossRef]
39. Springer, S.; Wang, Y.; Dal Molin, M.; Masica, D.L.; Jiao, Y.; Kinde, I.; Blackford, A.; Raman, S.P.; Wolfgang, C.L.; Tomita, T.; et al. A combination of molecular markers and clinical features improve the classification of pancreatic cysts. *Gastroenterology* **2015**, *149*, 1501–1510. [CrossRef]
40. Garbett, N.C.; Miller, J.J.; Jenson, A.B.; Miller, D.M.; Chaires, J.B. Interrogation of the plasma proteome with differential scanning calorimetry. *Clin. Chem.* **2007**, *53*, 2012–2014. [CrossRef]
41. Wiegand, N.; Bűcs, G.; Dandé, Á.; Lőrinczy, D. Investigation of protein content of synovial fluids with DSC in different arthritides. *J. Therm. Anal. Calorim.* **2019**. [CrossRef]
42. Brandts, J.F.; Lin, L.N. Study of strong to ultratight protein interactions using differential scanning calorimetry. *Biochemistry* **1990**, *29*, 6927–6940. [CrossRef] [PubMed]
43. Do, M.; Han, D.; Wang, J.I.; Kim, H.; Kwon, W.; Han, Y.; Jang, J.Y.; Kim, Y. Quantitative proteomic analysis of pancreatic cyst fluid proteins associated with malignancy in intraductal papillary mucinous neoplasms. *Clin. Proteom.* **2018**, *15*, 17. [CrossRef] [PubMed]
44. Ludwig, H.; Evstatiev, R.; Kornek, G.; Aapro, M.; Bauernhofer, T.; Buxhofer-Ausch, V.; Fridrik, M.; Geissler, D.; Geissler, K.; Gisslinger, H.; et al. Iron metabolism and iron supplementation in cancer patients. *Wien. Klin Wochenschr.* **2015**, *127*, 907–919. [CrossRef] [PubMed]
45. Forciniti, S.; Greco, L.; Grizzi, F.; Malesci, A.; Laghi, L. Iron Metabolism in Cancer Progression. *Int. J. Mol. Sci.* **2020**, *21*, 2257. [CrossRef] [PubMed]

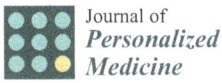

Journal of
Personalized
Medicine

Review

Defects in MMR Genes as a Seminal Example of Personalized Medicine: From Diagnosis to Therapy

Arianna Dal Buono [1], Federica Gaiani [2], Laura Poliani [1,3], Carmen Correale [1] and Luigi Laghi [2,4,*]

1 Division of Gastroenterology, Department of Gastroenterology, Humanitas Research Hospital—IRCCS, 20089 Rozzano, Italy; arianna.dalbuono@humanitas.it (A.D.B.); poliani.laura@hsr.it (L.P.); carmen.correale@humanitasresearch.it (C.C.)
2 Department of Medicine and Surgery, University of Parma, 43121 Parma, Italy; federica.gaiani@unipr.it
3 Gastroenterology and Endoscopy Unit, IRCCS Ospedale San Raffaele, 20132 Milan, Italy
4 Laboratory of Molecular Gastroenterology, Humanitas Research Hospital—IRCCS, 20089 Rozzano, Italy
* Correspondence: luigiandreagiuseppe.laghi@unipr.it

Abstract: Microsatellite instability (MSI) is the landmark feature of DNA mismatch repair deficiency, which can be found in 15–20% of all colorectal cancers (CRC). This specific set of tumors has been initially perceived as a niche for geneticists or gastroenterologists focused on inherited predispositions. However, over the years, MSI has established itself as a key biomarker for the diagnosis, then extending to forecasting the disease behavior and prognostication, including the prediction of responsiveness to immunotherapy and eventually to kinase inhibitors, and possibly even to specific biological drugs. Thanks to the contribution of the characterization of MSI tumors, researchers have first acknowledged that a strong lymphocytic reaction is associated with a good prognosis. This understanding supported the prognostic implications in terms of the low metastatic potential of MSI-CRC and has led to modifications in the indications for adjuvant treatment. Furthermore, with the emergence of immunotherapy, this strong biomarker of responsiveness has exemplified the capability of re-activating an effective immune control by removing the brakes of immune evasion. Lately, a subset of MSI-CRC emerged as the ideal target for kinase inhibitors. This therapeutic scenario implies a paradox in which appropriate treatments for advanced disease are effective in a set of tumors that seldom evolve towards metastases.

Keywords: microsatellite instability; colorectal cancer; immunotherapy; targeted therapy

Citation: Dal Buono, A.; Gaiani, F.; Poliani, L.; Correale, C.; Laghi, L. Defects in MMR Genes as a Seminal Example of Personalized Medicine: From Diagnosis to Therapy. *J. Pers. Med.* **2021**, *11*, 1333. https://doi.org/10.3390/jpm11121333

Academic Editors: Enrico Mini and Stefania Nobili

Received: 3 October 2021
Accepted: 6 December 2021
Published: 8 December 2021

Publisher's Note: MDPI stays neutral with regard to jurisdictional claims in published maps and institutional affiliations.

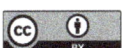

Copyright: © 2021 by the authors. Licensee MDPI, Basel, Switzerland. This article is an open access article distributed under the terms and conditions of the Creative Commons Attribution (CC BY) license (https://creativecommons.org/licenses/by/4.0/).

1. Introduction

Colorectal cancer (CRC) is the third most common malignancy and cause of cancer mortality in Europe and the United States, accounting for nearly 900.000 deaths every year worldwide [1]. Among the newly diagnosed CRC, approximately 20% of patients still present with a metastatic disease, and a further 25% of those with an initially localized disease will eventually develop distant metastases [2,3]. Despite the fact that staging has traditionally represented the backbone of the prognostic factors in oncology, the growing knowledge of the molecular mechanisms of CRC has revolutionized the traditional or "old school" methods of managing tumor conditions. Indeed, CRC is a highly heterogeneous disease in regard to molecular expression and genetic abnormalities. It is known that a small subset of CRCs, approximately 15% of the cases, demonstrate microsatellite instability (MSI) due to an impaired DNA mismatch repair (MMR) system, though the vast majority of CRCs belong to the microsatellite stable (MSS) biomarker list [4]. MSI-CRCs are mostly sporadic, while approximately 3% of all CRCs harbor a germline mutation of mismatch repair genes (i.e., *MLH1*, *MSH2*, *MSH6*, *PMS2*, and *EpCAM*) identifying the Lynch syndrome [5]. The understanding of the carcinogenesis of MMR deficient tumors and subsequent clinical research has had an enormous therapeutic impact in the field of gastrointestinal oncology. In particular, the MSI status defines the largest group of inherited predispositions to gastrointestinal cancers and impacts the prognosis of CRC, giving better stage-adjusted survival rates compared to MSS tumors [6,7]. Moreover, MSI colorectal tumors are more frequently seen at early stages (i.e., stage II–III), and only 3.5% of the cases present with a metastatic disease [8], in accordance with a reduced distant metastasis, which is intrinsic to MSI status. MMR/MSI testing is increasingly being incorporated as a standard of care for all CRC patients and is collectively recommended by the most important scientific societies involved in the field, such as AGA, ASGE, ASCRS, ASCO, and ESMO [9]. This review summarizes the evidence demonstrating the value of MSI as a diagnostic and prognostic tool and eventually also a predictive biomarker in the personalized approach to CRC.

2. Discovery of MSI, Its Relevance in Lynch Syndrome and Understanding the Different Molecular Pathogenesis of CRC

2.1. Parallel Discovery

The discovery of DNA mismatch repair (MMR) defects is an interesting outcome, which testifies how the contemporary efforts of different teams have helped to elucidate the molecular basis of Lynch syndrome (LS) in a relatively short period of time. However, in addition to contributing to the development of a new era in molecular medicine, it has also raised other lessons in LS management that are worth recalling. The reason for this is chiefly that different methodological approaches were used by the groups involved in the research. To be precise, finding the mechanism behind LS was not the shared aim of these teams. The study led by Perucho was involved in identifying a particular mechanism of carcinogenesis through an unbiased molecular approach, defined as an "arbitrarily primed polymerase chain reaction" (PCR) [10,11]. In doing so, his group found that a fraction of CRCs harbored un-corrected frame-shifted DNA tracts, and they referred to such changes as ubiquitous somatic mutations. The team led by Thibodeau [12] was looking for allelic losses (and gains) by PCR and noted that there was "instability" at the amplified microsatellite sequences (hence microsatellite instability or MSI), in some proportion of the CRCs. Neither study was familiar with or looking for familial cancer or Lynch syndrome genes. Meanwhile, an international consortium with a strong membership from Finland, including Aaltonen, was trying to identify the loci associated with Lynch syndrome by employing an allelotyping approach to search for loss of heterozygosity [13,14]. With the exploration of dinucleotide repeats in tumor DNA compared to normal subjects, CRC patients were found to have frame-shifted sequences, which they described as replication errors (RER). Subsequently, the term MSI was used to describe the same phenomenon that these groups identified and described, although the degree of competition was very high. Perucho's reference to a probable inherited syndrome was incorporated within the manuscript after Aaltonen and Vogelstein's group had mapped and reported a Lynch syndrome locus on 2p, a finding already detected by Perucho. In a timely editorial, it was noted that "the cancers whose cells carry shortened repeats are differently distributed in the colon from others and metastasize less frequently. If Perucho is right in believing that the underlying fault may be a mutation of a DNA repair gene, the ramifications of that may be exceedingly important" [15]. These words summarized the relevant biological and clinical implications of the discovery of DNA MMR defects.

These inherent differences led to a dual development of research efforts in the field. On one side, the genes involved in DNA mismatch repair in humans were targeted, being first identified by Kolodner [16] and subsequently largely addressed in their relevance by various teams, including that led by Bert Vogelstein [17], as part of his landmark work unravelling the molecular bases of CRC, before and after the discovery of MMR defects.

On the other side, the research focused on the molecular pathogenesis of MMR deficient CRC and addressed the role of these types of mutations in the peculiar behavior of MSI tumors. It soon became evident that these cancers remain in a class of their own among tumors [18], as compared to other known genetic pathways to CRC, mainly driven by *APC* gene damage both in inherited (i.e., Familial Adenomatous Polyposis) and sporadic carcinogenesis. In this respect, MMR-deficient tumors appear mainly a disease marked by accelerated tumor progression rather than by an accelerated tumor initiation. It was appreciated that the burden of unrepaired mutations in these tumors contributes to their indolent behavior [19,20] and to the amount of immune response that they elicit [21,22]. Surprisingly, these areas of investigation took years to generate translational research aimed at systematically identifying prognostic markers for CRC and then influencing clinical practice. It should be mentioned that for the first time since the discovery of MMR defects and MSI, a molecular phenotype has recently been proposed for the molecular screening of a specific disease subtype [23]. This long journey led to the exclusion from adjuvant therapy of patients with stage IIA MSI CRC, even though they displayed high-risk hallmarks and contributed to defining the role of tumor-infiltrating lymphocytes (TILs) as a prognostic marker in CRC staging (see below).

2.2. Unraveling the Pool of Genes Involved in DNA MMR and Deranged in Lynch Syndrome

MMR is a mechanism whereby proteins identify and repair mismatched bases occurring mostly by statistical chance during DNA replication or genetic recombination, a mechanism that is present among many species. DNA mismatching, however, is also enhanced by chemical or physical damage. The high conservation rate among species accounts for its importance, as does the discovery of its involvement in human disease by a basic scientist [16]. He was able to cross its defects with the by-then emerging phenotype of MSI in human CRC, thus developing a strategy to identify one of its components (namely, *MSH2*) as the culprit for a fraction of the cases of Lynch syndrome, moving from the similarities of molecular signatures in yeasts. That is why the human genes were initially labelled as homologues of their counterpart in yeasts.

As the result of a plurality of efforts, we now know that this system is constituted by multiple proteins, including MLH1 (MutL homologue), PMS2 (post-meiotic segregation protein), MSH2 (MutS homologue), MSH6, MLH3, MSH3, and PMS1, which form heterodimers with different roles: MSH2/MSH6 and MSH2/MSH3 heterodimers recognize and bind base–base mismatches and insertion/deletion loops, and subsequently, they recruit MLH1/PMS2 heterodimers to excise and allow the resynthesis of corrected strands [4,24,25]. Later, deletions of the 3′ distal portion of the *EPCAM* gene, containing the termination codon, have been demonstrated to influence the MMR system by leading to the methylation of the promoter of the downstream neighbor *MSH2* and therein to its silencing [26]. Genetic or epigenetic events leading to the silencing of one of the genes of the MMR system ensues in the appearance of the mutator phenotype. Irrespective of the underlying molecular mechanisms, the inactivation of any of the members of the MMR genes leads to the disappearance of the encoded protein. However, the loss of MSH2 or MLH1 also leads to the loss of expression of that protein itself and its heterodimer partner, whereas the loss of MSH6 or PMS2 results in the loss of expression only of the specific protein. Accordingly, germline inactivating mutations of the genes encoding for one among the MMR proteins stay at the basis of MSI as the first pathogenetic damage of the Lynch syndrome and should be followed by a second somatic inactivation hit according to the Knudson hypothesis turning off the second allele [24,27].

In the seminal phase of the late 1990s, addressing MSI in clinical practice was mostly based on clinical criteria, namely the Bethesda ones [28,29]. In other words, the clinical criteria used to define Lynch syndrome (by then referred to as Hereditary Non-Polyposis CRC, HNPCC) or Amsterdam criteria [30,31] were loosened and expanded to identify those patients suitable for the analysis of the MS-status of their CRC and then to germline sequencing if the results of the somatic analysis revealed MSI. Initially, the characterizations of tumor samples based on MS-status comprised the classification into microsatellite instability high (MSI-H) if two or more of the microsatellite markers show instability (or >30% of unstable markers if a larger panel is used) and microsatellite instability low (MSI-L) if only one marker shows instability, as opposed to MSS cancers [24,32]. However, such a classification has been variably criticized, and the distinction in MSI-H and MSI-L progressively lost relevance, and the latter group is cumulated with MSS tumors [33,34].

The systematization of the characterization of the MS status in CRC has confirmed the initial findings by Perucho et al. that most MSI tumors are not the epiphenomenon of LS but are instead sporadic. In fact, considering that MSI cancers account for 15% of all CRCs, only 3% of the total (or 20% among MSI cases) are attributable to Lynch syndrome [35]. It is also now clear that hereditary MSI cancers differ from sporadic ones by means of the type of underlying alteration causing the impairment of the MMR system (as well as in their clinical behavior).

2.3. Sporadic MSI Cancers and Hypermethylation

Patients with sporadic MSI CRC are significantly older than those affected by Lynch syndrome, and most of them lack any significant familial clustering, nevertheless maintaining a better prognosis than those with MSS tumors [36]. The molecular features of sporadic MSI tumors, instead of germline pathogenic variants of MMR genes plus second hit on the other allele, are the methylation of *MLH1* promoter frequently coupled with the mutation *BRAF*(V600E) [4,37].

Understanding the molecular pathogenesis of sporadic MSI CRC was the sequel of the discovery of germline MMR defects, which has helped clarify the mechanism for a portion of otherwise unexplained cases, as well as introducing one additional cancer phenotype [38–40]. In fact, the main mechanism for a sporadic MSI CRC going through the inactivation of the promoter region of the DNA mismatch repair gene *MLH1* by hypermethylation [41] mostly occurs in the context of the CpG island methylator phenotype (CIMP) [42]. CpG islands are genomic regions rich in cytosine and guanine repeats present in about 40–50% of human genes, usually located at the promoter region and crucial for the epigenetic inactivation of gene transcription by hypermethylation [42].

Although the methylator phenotype can be intended as the main molecular biomarker of sporadic MSI tumors, CIMP can also be found in a group of patients who present no anomalies of the MMR system. Further studies by Ogino et al. [43] and Samowitz et al. [44] demonstrated that not all sporadic MSI tumors with *MLH1* hypermethylation have a methylator phenotype. The scenario of CRC molecular characterization has become more and more complex over the years, adding the CIMP status as a separate parameter of classification [41,45]. CIMP+ (or CIMP-high) CRCs are reported to be more frequent in the elderly and in women, are often located in the proximal location, show poor differentiation, and have a high frequency of MSI and *BRAF* mutation [41,46,47], largely overlapping with sporadic MSI cases. CIMP was originally described as the *de novo* methylation of the 5′ CpG island of p16 (now *CDNK2A*) detectable in approximately 1/5 of different tumor types and acting as an alternative mechanism for the silencing of tumor suppressor genes [48].

Although the value of CIMP is not well known, CIMP+ CRC seems to have a better outcome than CIMP-low (particularly if showing wild-type *BRAF*) and appears to respond more efficiently to adjuvant treatments [41].

2.4. Lynch Syndrome versus Lynch-Like Syndrome

The seminal report on what will be later referred to as HNPCC and Lynch syndrome dates to the end of the XIX century by Aldred S. Warthin, who reported the pedigree of "family G" with a cluster of uterine, gastric, and abdominal cancer, which led him to suspect the existence of a form of predisposition [49]. Years later, Henry Lynch reported similar familial clusters of cancer and reviewed the history of family G, with a predominance of cancers of the colon, uterus and stomach [50]. Notably, Lynch concluded the culprit was an autosomal dominant inheritance of this otherwise unrecognized syndromic cluster, referred to as "Cancer Family Syndrome" (for an exhaustive perspective on the historical development of the medical perspective on the topic, see Boland, 2013) [50]. Later, the term HNPCC was used to refer to the lack of a phenotypic hallmark compared to polyposis syndromes [51]. However, once a molecular phenotype had been identified and its basis clarified, the term Lynch syndrome was encouraged and adopted for those cases with a defined MMR defect and a germline mutation in the MMR genes. Alternately, the lack of a pathogenic germline mutation in a patient with an MSI CRC and features suggestive of an underlying predisposition is called "Lynch-like" syndrome [52,53]. The two syndromes have the development of MSI CRCs at a young age and the presence of extracolonic cancers in common. However, although in patients affected by Lynch-like syndrome, the onset of cancer is in the fifth decade (mean age, 54.9 years) [53], the standardized incidence ratios of CRC and extracolonic cancers is lower (2.12 vs. 6.04 and 1.69 vs. 2.81, respectively) [54].

Although Lynch-like syndrome patients lack germline mutations of the MMR system, they exhibit in almost half of all cases the biallelic somatic inactivation of DNA MMR genes within the tumor [54,55]; moreover, they might harbor germline mutations of unknown genes other than MMR ones. Nevertheless, due to the increased cancer risk for the proband and his or her relatives, a careful follow-up remains advisable from a clinical perspective [54,55].

3. Prognostic Value of MSI in CRC

3.1. Lower Metastatic Potential and Better Survival of MSI CRC

MSI is undoubtedly a positive prognostic factor in CRC patients, which is promptly explained by the low prevalence of MSI tumors among metastatic CRCs, corresponding to 2–4% of stage IV cases [4,25], as compared to their prevalence in earlier stages [56,57]. MSI CRCs typically present a dense immune cell infiltration, particularly rich in TILs, which has been associated with a better prognosis and a reduced tendency to metastasize [8]. Substantial evidence supports that MSI is a strong prognostic marker in early-stage CRCs with a favorable impact on survival, beyond the TNM staging system also from pooled retrospective analyses [58]. With respect to stage II CRC patients, in the ACCENT database analysis, the MSI profile significantly improved the disease-free survival and the overall survival [59].

Compared to stage II, the prognostic value of MSI in stage III CRC is less defined, and contradictory data have emerged from randomized clinical trials (RCTs) and meta-analysis [60–62] (see below).

Summarizing the available data, MSI confers a favorable prognosis in stage II CRC, and this effect seems to be progressively reduced with advancing stage (i.e., stage III) [60–62]. A speculative explanation of this phenomenon lies in the evasion of immune surveillance that is possibly acquired in more advanced stages of the disease. In accordance with the above statement, in stage IV CRCs, MSI no longer provides an advantage in terms of prognosis [63,64], though interactions with chemotherapy, as the standard adjuvant treatment for stage III CRC, should not be disregarded despite being difficult to disentangle.

3.2. Adaptive Immune Response and the Relevance of Immune Parameters

MSI-CRCs attract a dense lymphocytic infiltrate [21,22], parallelly driving the infiltration of specific subsets of immune cells (i.e., cytotoxic and helper T-lymphocytes) that are associated with an improved prognosis and reduced recurrence rates after surgery [63], especially in patients with early, node-negative CRC, largely contributing to the prognostic advantage of high densities of infiltrating lymphocytes [65].

Among the immune subpopulations recruited by MSI-CRC, dendritic cells and T cells activate the immune antitumoral response, which is downstream accomplished by activated memory CD4 + T cells, NK cells, M1 macrophages, and neutrophils [66]. The attempt to measure the immune infiltrate in the primary tumor and to assess its prognostic value has been pursued by trying to build a reliable "immuno-score" that quantifies the amount of infiltrating T-lymphocytes and allows inferences on CRC outcomes [67]. The immuno-score has been suggested to be superior to the conventional TNM classification in CRC, given its ability to differentiate patients with a better or worse prognosis in MSS and MSI disease, as across the various stages according to AJCC/UICC [68]. The measure of CD8+ cells and CD45RO+ memory cells in specific tumor regions (i.e., at the invasive front) has been, in fact, linked to longer overall survival in MSI-CRC patients [69]. This parameter is likely to be included in the TNM staging, similarly to its use for MSI, although some refinement is necessary in order to better define its reliability in stage III disease [36,44].

4. Predictive Value of MSI

4.1. Implication for the Adjuvant Treatment: Stage 2 vs. Stage 3

In stage II CRC, MSI has been endorsed as a reliable predictive indicator associated with a lack of benefit from adjuvant chemotherapy (5-fluorouracil-based (5FU)). This clinical endorsement first moved from the better prognosis and lower metastatic potential of MSI CRCs [56,57].

The initial report on non-responsiveness came from a study by Ribic et al. in which patients with MSI CRC were found to have a better overall 5-year survival, especially when not receiving adjuvant chemotherapy [70]. Subsequently, Sargent, in a collaborative study, confirmed this finding by showing that MSI interacted significantly with chemotherapy and that there was no improvement in patients with stage II MSI CRC who had received 5-FU [71]. Sinicrope et al. shortly after confirmed that patients with MSI CRC have lower rates of tumor recurrence, delayed time to relapse, and improved survival rates, with respect to MSS CRC patients [72]. Adjuvant treatment also reduced the rate of distant recurrences in patients with stage III CRC, which could be significant in patients with germline pathogenic variants compared to those with sporadic tumors [73].

A milestone in modern oncology was placed in the phase III Quick and Simple and Reliable (QUASAR) trial that randomized more than 2000 patients affected by stage II CRC to either receive adjuvant chemotherapy with 5-FU or for observation [74]. The study showed a significantly reduced risk of recurrence for MMR-deficient CRC (risk ratio, 0.53, 95% C.I., 0.40–0.70; $p < 0.001$) as compared to proficient ones, and the subanalysis for MMR status demonstrated no benefit from adjuvant chemotherapy [74]. This evidence has been confirmed by several meta-analyses that established MSI status as a predictive factor for both therapy response and relapse rates as concerns in stage II CRC [75–77]. Overall, data support MSI as the leading molecular marker with clinical value in early-stage CRC; no further molecular stigma has been incorporated in the management algorithms of CRC yet.

The situation in stage III appears more complex. In a study on patients included in a randomized trial on adjuvant 5-FU plus Oxaliplatin and folinic acid (FOLFOX) after resection of stage III CRC, Sinicrope et al. found that *KRAS* and *BRAF* mutations had a negative prognostic effect on disease-free survival, while MSI was not prognostic in all patients but significantly interacted with the tumor site and nodal status [78]. Accordingly, only patients with right-sided MSI CRC had a better outcome, and such an advantage was lost in those with N2 tumors [78].

In an interesting study assessing the value of lymphocyte infiltration in patients included in the PETACC8 phase III study [79], the authors found that MSI was not a predictive factor for overall survival in treated patients [79]. However, a larger study adding patients from the NCCTG N0147 trial [80] found that patients with MMR-deficient CRCs had significantly longer disease-free survival than those with proficient tumors at multivariate analyses (HR, 0.73; 95% CI, 0.54–0.97; $p = 0.03$), although such advantage may become evident only after 18 months at Kaplan–Meier survival curves. One issue involves the benefit of oxaliplatin added to 5-flurouracil [80]. Interestingly, it had been shown earlier that in an MSH2-deficient mouse model developing CRC, FOLFOX treatment led to a reduction in tumor volume, and MMR status was found not to modify responsiveness to oxaliplatin in previous studies [81,82].

Other studies further clarified that *KRAS* and *BRAF* mutations act as negative prognostic factors in MSS CRC patients treated with adjuvant FOLFOX, but not in MSI patients [83].

4.2. Removing the Breaks from the Immune Response: Immunotherapy

In the last decade, translational research in oncology has been focusing on the molecular mechanisms driving the interaction between MSI CRC and the immune system. The MSI status influences the tumoral microenvironment and the interactions with the immune system through multiple aspects, therefore impacting the efficacy of immunotherapy. A defective MMR leads to a high tumor mutational burden (TMB) [11,19,20], which means that tumoral cells profusely generate highly immunogenic soluble and surface neoantigens able to attract cytotoxic and helper T-lymphocytes [22,84]. The higher somatic mutational load that increases the presentation of neoepitopes has been epitomized as one of the mediators of the observed augmented response to immunotherapy as well in MSI tumors [85,86]. The immunogenicity of these neoantigens, structurally frame-shifted peptides, lies in their ability to bind with major histocompatibility complex class I (MHC-I) alleles [87]. Moreover, the neo-antigen load was directly associated with the T-cell memory tumoral infiltration [87].

Secondly, as demonstrated by Llosa et al., neoplastic cells with MMR defect overexpress several immune checkpoint proteins (e.g., PD-1, PD-L1, CTLA-4, LAG-3, and IDO), compared to MSS cancers [88].

These findings, together with evidence stemming from clinical trials, initially led immune checkpoint inhibitors (i.e., anti-PD1) to be approved by the regulatory authorities exclusively according to the MSI status, regardless of cancer type [8].

Recent studies investigating anti-programmed death-1 (PD-1) checkpoint inhibitors have identified and demonstrated MS status as a biomarker predictive of therapy response [89,90]. MMR-deficient cancers are now acknowledged to be sensitive to anti-PD1 (nivolumab, pembrolizumab) with or without anti-cytotoxic T-lymphocyte-associated protein 4 (CTLA-4) antibodies [89,90].

4.3. Silencing Map Kinases in Sporadic MSI

In the current landscape, it has become clear that *BRAF*-mutant CRC represents a distinct biologic entity, typically refractory to the traditional chemotherapy regimens [91]. *BRAF* is a serine/threonine kinase that acts downstream of *KRAS* in the mitogen-activated protein kinase (MAPK) cellular signaling pathway. *BRAF*-mutant CRC commonly exhibits a valine to glutamic-acid variation, specifically at codon 600 (V600E; or 1799T>A). The effect of this change is a constitutively activated protein. The *BRAF* V600E mutation overlaps with sporadic MSI-CRC in up to 33% of the cases [92].

Historically, *BRAF*-mutated CRCs have been associated with a significantly worse prognosis [93]. The therapeutic implications of targeting this mutation came as a lesson from the management of *BRAF*-mutated melanomas, and currently, several ongoing clinical trials are investigating the efficacy of BRAF-inhibitors (i.e., dabrafenib, vemurafenib, or encorafenib) alone or in combination in patients with metastatic *BRAF* (V600E)-mutated CRC [94].

In terms of personalized medicine, the inhibition of MAPK signaling in sporadic MSI-CRCs has been explored with promising results. In a pivotal, single-arm study that included 43 patients with *BRAF*-V600E metastatic CRC treated with the adjunct of a MEK inhibitor (Trametinib), the results showed improved response rates compared with BRAF inhibition alone [95]. A further phase II study, comparing dabrafenib, trametinib, and panitumumab triple therapy with double therapies (either dabrafenib plus panitumumab or trametinib plus panitumumab), assessed a disease control rate (response and stable disease together) in 86% of patients [96]. The median progression-free survival (PFS) and the duration of response were 4.2 and 7.6 months, respectively [96].

Based on these preliminary data, the combination therapies of BRAF/MEK have not been approved by the Food and Drug Administration (FDA) for the treatment of metastatic *BRAF* V600E CRC yet. Lastly, clinical trials examining immunotherapy in combination with inhibitors of the MAPK pathway are expected.

5. Discussion and Concluding Remarks

This review illustrates the current evidence on the prognostic and predictive value of MSI as a trail maker of the personalized medicine approach to CRC. Compared to MSS CRC, MSI status is associated with a more favorable prognosis in early-stage CRCs [58].

Furthermore, based on the evidence that adjuvant chemotherapy does not add any advantage for the prognosis in stage II, knowledge of MSI status drives clinical decisions for these patients [59]. Conversely, the prognostic value of MSI with respect to stage III disease appears attenuated, and these patients are, so far, recommended to receive standard adjuvant chemotherapy.

Regarding the predictive value of MSI status, it has been extensively demonstrated to be a robust biomarker for a good response to immune checkpoint inhibitors in patients with metastatic disease [89,90]. However, the precise role of immunotherapy in earlier-stage CRCs needs to be clarified by ongoing randomized studies. The studies on the molecular heterogeneity and tumoral microenvironment surrounding MSI tumors have led to an increased understanding of possible innovative therapeutic targets.

Figure 1 summarizes the timeline of the gradual achievement of a progressively wider clinical usefulness of MSI status in the field of CRC.

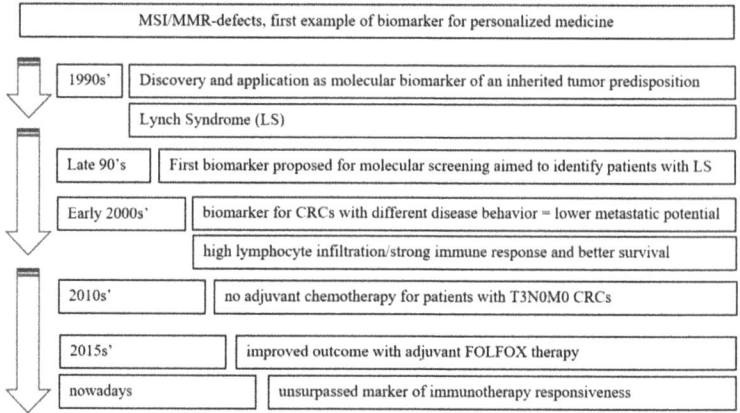

Figure 1. MMR story: lessons from a long-lasting biomarker. Timeline of its gradual achievement of wider clinical usefulness.

Finally, research has recently been focusing on the relationship between gut microbiota and CRC tumorigenesis, with a particular interest in the induced molecular profile, such as MSI. What is emerging is that, among the different microbiological species, *Fusobacterium nucleatum* is linked to the development of MSI tumors [97,98]. Indeed, tumors with high levels of *Fusobacterium nucleatum* tend to occur in the proximal colon and have a higher incidence of MSI with rather poor survival, as reported in a prospective cohort study [98]. This seems somehow counterintuitive, and it has been associated with the capability of *Fusobacterium nucleatum* to suppress the adaptive immune response in MSI-CRCs [99].

In the foreseeable future, gut bacterial modulation or a fecal microbiota transplant could stimulate the immune response in patients with MSI-CRCs that have developed a secondary resistance to immunotherapy. Thus, the modulation of the microbiota and increased antigen presentation appear to be two possible therapeutic targets for new and personalized strategies aimed, for example, at restoring a competent immune response and immunotherapy efficacy in MSI tumors. As we have gleaned much more than we would have expected from the MSI tumor subtype, we should be confident there is yet more to learn.

T3N0M0 CRCs, or stage IIA, invade through the muscularis propria into the subserosa but have not reached nearby organs and lymph nodes and have not spread to distant organs [100]. FOLFOX, comprising of 5-FU, Oxaliplatin, and Folinic acid, is administered after surgery as adjuvant treatment.

Author Contributions: Conceptualization, L.L.; methodology, A.D.B., F.G.; writing—original draft preparation, A.D.B., F.G.; writing—review and editing, L.P. and C.C.; supervision, L.L. All authors have read and agreed to the published version of the manuscript.

Funding: This research received no external funding.

Institutional Review Board Statement: Not applicable.

Informed Consent Statement: Not applicable.

Conflicts of Interest: The authors declare no conflict of interest.

Abbreviations

CRC	colorectal carcinoma
MMR	mismatch repair
MSI	microsatellite instability
LS	Lynch syndrome
TILs	tumor-infiltrating lymphocytes

References

1. Biller, L.H.; Schrag, D. Diagnosis and Treatment of Metastatic Colorectal Cancer: A Review. *JAMA* **2021**, *325*, 669–685. [CrossRef] [PubMed]
2. Siegel, R.L.; Miller, K.D.; Goding Sauer, A.; Fedewa, S.A.; Butterly, L.F.; Anderson, J.C.; Cercek, A.; Smith, R.A.; Jemal, A. Colorectal cancer statistics, 2020. *CA Cancer J. Clin.* **2020**, *70*, 145–164. [CrossRef]
3. National Cancer Institute Surveillance, Epidemiology, and End Results Program. Cancer Stat Facts: Colorectal Cancer. Available online: https://seer.cancer.gov/statfacts/html/colorect.html (accessed on 9 September 2021).
4. Boland, C.R.; Goel, A. Microsatellite instability in colorectal cancer. *Gastroenterology* **2010**, *138*, 2073–2087. [CrossRef]
5. Ward, R.; Meagher, A.; Tomlinson, I.; O'Connor, T.; Norrie, M.; Wu, R.; Hawkins, N. Microsatellite instability and the clinico-pathological features of sporadic colorectal cancer. *Gut* **2001**, *48*, 821–882. [CrossRef] [PubMed]
6. Taieb, J.; Shi, Q.; Pederson, L.; Alberts, S.; Wolmark, N.; Van Cutsem, E.; de Gramont, A.; Kerr, R.; Grothey, A.; Lonardi, S.; et al. Prognosis of microsatellite instability and/or mismatch repair deficiency stage III colon cancer patients after disease recurrence following adjuvant treatment: Results of an ACCENT pooled analysis of seven studies. *Ann. Oncol.* **2019**, *30*, 1466–1471. [CrossRef] [PubMed]
7. Jin, Z.; Sinicrope, F.A. Prognostic and Predictive Values of Mismatch Repair Deficiency in Non-Metastatic Colorectal Cancer. *Cancers* **2021**, *13*, 300. [CrossRef]
8. Ganesh, K.; Stadler, Z.K.; Cercek, A.; Mendelsohn, R.B.; Shia, J.; Segal, N.H.; Diaz, L.A., Jr. Immunotherapy in colorectal cancer: Rationale, challenges and potential. *Nat. Rev. Gastroenterol. Hepatol.* **2019**, *16*, 361–375. [CrossRef] [PubMed]
9. Messersmith, W.A. NCCN Guidelines Updates: Management of Metastatic Colorectal Cancer. *J. Natl. Compr. Canc. Net.* **2019**, *17*, 599–601.
10. Peinado, M.A.; Malkhosyan, S.; Velazquez, A.; Perucho, M. Isolation and characterization of allelic losses and gains in colorectal tumors by arbitrarily primed polymerase chain reaction. *Proc. Natl. Acad. Sci. USA* **1992**, *89*, 10065–10069. [CrossRef]
11. Ionov, Y.; Peinado, M.A.; Malkhosyan, S.; Shibata, D.; Perucho, M. Ubiquitous somatic mutations in simple repeated sequences reveal a new mechanism for colonic carcinogenesis. *Nature* **1993**, *363*, 558–561. [CrossRef]
12. Thibodeau, S.N.; Bren, G.; Schaid, D. Microsatellite Instability in Cancer of the Proximal Colon. *Science* **1993**, *260*, 816–819. [CrossRef] [PubMed]
13. Aaltonen, L.A.; Peltomäki, P.; Leach, F.S.; Sistonen, P.; Pylkkänen, L.; Mecklin, J.-P.; Järvinen, H.; Powell, S.M.; Jen, J.; Hamilton, S.R.; et al. Clues to the Pathogenesis of Familial Colorectal Cancer. *Science* **1993**, *260*, 812–816. [CrossRef] [PubMed]
14. Peltomäki, P.; Aaltonen, L.A.; Sistonen, P.; Pylkkänen, L.; Mecklin, J.-P.; Järvinen, H.; Green, J.S.; Jass, J.R.; Weber, J.L.; Leach, F.S.; et al. Genetic Mapping of a Locus Predisposing to Human Colorectal Cancer. *Science* **1993**, *260*, 810–812. [CrossRef]
15. Maddox, J. Competition and the death of science. *Nature* **1993**, *363*, 667. [CrossRef]
16. Fishel, R.; Lescoe, M.K.; Rao, M.R.; Copeland, N.G.; Jenkins, N.A.; Garber, J.; Kane, M.; Kolodner, R. The human mutator gene homolog MSH2 and its association with hereditary nonpolyposis colon cancer. *Cell* **1993**, *75*, 1027–1038. [CrossRef]
17. Leach, F.S.; Nicolaides, N.C.; Papadopoulos, N.; Liu, B.; Jen, J.; Parsons, R.; Peltomäki, P.; Sistonen, P.; Aaltonen, L.; Nyström-Lahti, M.; et al. Mutations of a mutS homolog in hereditary nonpolyposis colorectal cancer. *Cell* **1993**, *75*, 1215–1225. [CrossRef]
18. Kinzler, K.W.; Vogelstein, B. Lessons from Hereditary Colorectal Cancer. *Cell* **1996**, *87*, 159–170. [CrossRef]
19. Malkhosyan, S.; Rampino, N.; Yamamoto, H.; Perucho, M. Frameshift mutator mutations. *Nature* **1996**, *382*, 499–500. [CrossRef] [PubMed]
20. Perucho, M. Microsatellite instability: The mutator that mutates the other mutator. *Nat. Med.* **1996**, *2*, 630–631. [CrossRef] [PubMed]

21. Kim, H.; Jen, J.; Vogelstein, B.; Hamilton, S.R. Clinical and pathological characteristics of sporadic colorectal carcinomas with DNA replication errors in microsatellite sequences. *Am. J. Pathol.* **1994**, *145*, 148–156. [PubMed]
22. Guidoboni, M.; Gafà, R.; Viel, A.; Doglioni, C.; Russo, A.; Santini, A.; Del Tin, L.; Macrì, E.; Lanza, G.; Boiocchi, M.; et al. Microsatellite instability and high content of activated cytotoxic lymphocytes identify colon cancer patients with a favorable prognosis. *Am. J. Pathol.* **2001**, *159*, 297–304. [CrossRef]
23. Aaltonen, L.A.; Salovaara, R.; Kristo, P.; Canzian, F.; Hemminki, A.; Peltomäki, P.; Chadwick, R.B.; Kääriäinen, H.; Eskelinen, M.; Järvinen, H.; et al. Incidence of hereditary nonpolyposis colorectal cancer and the feasibility of molecular screening for the disease. *N. Engl. J. Med.* **1998**, *338*, 1481–1487. [CrossRef] [PubMed]
24. De' Angelis, G.L.; Bottarelli, L.; Azzoni, C.; De'Angelis, N.; Leandro, G.; Di Mario, F.; Gaiani, F.; Negri, F. Microsatellite instability in colorectal cancer. *Acta Biomed.* **2018**, *89*, 97–101.
25. Peltomäki, P. Update on Lynch syndrome genomics. *Fam. Cancer* **2016**, *15*, 385–393. [CrossRef]
26. Tutlewska, K.; Lubinski, J.; Kurzawski, G. Germline deletions in the EPCAM gene as a cause of Lynch syndrome—Literature review. *Hered. Cancer Clin. Pr.* **2013**, *11*, 9. [CrossRef] [PubMed]
27. Jiricny, J. The multifaceted mismatch-repair system. *Nat. Rev. Mol. Cell Biol.* **2006**, *7*, 335–346. [CrossRef] [PubMed]
28. Boland, C.R.; Thibodeau, S.N.; Hamilton, S.R.; Sidransky, D.; Eshleman, J.R.; Burt, R.W.; Meltzer, S.J.; Rodriguez-Bigas, M.A.; Fodde, R.; Ranzani, G.N.; et al. A National Cancer Institute Workshop on Microsatellite Instability for cancer detection and familial predisposition: Development of international criteria for the determination of microsatellite instability in colorectal cancer. *Cancer Res.* **1998**, *58*, 5248–5257. [PubMed]
29. Umar, A.; Boland, C.R.; Terdiman, J.P.; Syngal, S.; Chapelle, A.D.L.; Rüschoff, J.; Srivastava, S. Revised Bethesda Guidelines for hereditary nonpolyposis colorectal cancer (Lynch syndrome) and microsatellite instability. *J. Natl. Cancer Inst.* **2004**, *96*, 261–268. [CrossRef] [PubMed]
30. Vasen, H.F.; Mecklin, J.P.; Khan, P.M.; Lynch, H.T. The International Collaborative Group on Hereditary Non-Polyposis Colorectal Cancer (ICG-HNPCC). *Dis. Colon Rectum* **1991**, *34*, 424–425. [CrossRef]
31. Vasen, H.F.; Watson, P.; Mecklin, J.P.; Lynch, H.T. New clinical criteria for hereditary nonpolyposis colorectal cancer (HNPCC, Lynch syndrome) proposed by the International Collaborative group on HNPCC. *Gastroenterology* **1999**, *116*, 1453–1456. [CrossRef]
32. Jass, J.R. HNPCC and sporadic MSI-H colorectal cancer: A review of the morphological similarities and differences. *Fam Cancer* **2004**, *3*, 93–100. [CrossRef] [PubMed]
33. Laiho, P.; Launonen, V.; Lahermo, P.; Esteller, M.; Guo, M.; Herman, J.G.; Mecklin, J.P.; Järvinen, H.; Sistonen, P.; Kim, K.M.; et al. Low-level microsatellite instability in most colorectal carcinomas. *Cancer Res.* **2002**, *62*, 1166–1170.
34. Tomlinson, I.; Halford, S.; Aaltonen, L.; Hawkins, N.; Ward, R. Does MSI-low exist? *J. Pathol.* **2002**, *197*, 6–13. [CrossRef] [PubMed]
35. Hampel, H.; Frankel, W.L.; Martin, E.; Arnold, M.; Khanduja, K.; Kuebler, P.; Nakagawa, H.; Sotamaa, K.; Prior, T.W.; Westman, J.; et al. Screening for the Lynch syndrome (hereditary nonpolyposis colorectal cancer). *N. Engl. J. Med.* **2005**, *352*, 1851–1860. [CrossRef] [PubMed]
36. Laghi, L.; Negri, F.; Gaiani, F.; Cavalleri, T.; Grizzi, F.; De' Angelis, G.L.; Malesci, A. Prognostic and Predictive Cross-Roads of Microsatellite Instability and Immune Response to Colon Cancer. *Int. J. Mol. Sci.* **2020**, *21*, 9680. [CrossRef] [PubMed]
37. Domingo, E.; Laiho, P.; Ollikainen, M.; Pinto, M.; Wang, L.; French, A.J.; Westra, J.; Frebourg, T.; Espín, E.; Armengol, M.; et al. BRAF screening as a low-cost effective strategy for simplifying HNPCC genetic testing. *J. Med. Genet.* **2004**, *41*, 664–668. [CrossRef] [PubMed]
38. Kane, M.F.; Loda, M.; Gaida, G.M.; Lipman, J.; Mishra, R.; Goldman, H.; Jessup, J.M.; Kolodner, R. Methylation of the hMLH1 promoter correlates with lack of expression of hMLH1 in sporadic colon tumors and mismatch repair-defective human tumor cell lines. *Cancer Res.* **1997**, *57*, 808–811. [PubMed]
39. Cunningham, J.M.; Christensen, E.R.; Tester, D.J.; Kim, C.Y.; Roche, P.C.; Burgart, L.J.; Thibodeau, S.N. Hypermethylation of the hMLH1 promoter in colon cancer with microsatellite instability. *Cancer Res.* **1998**, *58*, 3455–3460.
40. Herman, J.G.; Umar, A.; Polyak, K.; Graff, J.R.; Ahuja, N.; Issa, J.P.; Markowitz, S.; Willson, J.K.; Hamilton, S.R.; Kinzler, K.W.; et al. Incidence and functional consequences of hMLH1 promoter hypermethylation in colorectal carcinoma. *Proc. Natl. Acad. Sci. USA* **1998**, *95*, 6870–6875. [CrossRef]
41. Gallois, C.; Laurent-Puig, P.; Taieb, J. Methylator phenotype in colorectal cancer: A prognostic factor or not? *Crit. Rev. Oncol. Hematol.* **2016**, *99*, 74–80. [CrossRef]
42. Toyota, M.; Ahuja, N.; Ohe-Toyota, M.; Herman, J.G.; Baylin, S.B.; Issa, J.-P. CpG island methylator phenotype in colorectal cancer. *Proc. Natl. Acad. Sci. USA* **1999**, *96*, 8681–8686. [CrossRef] [PubMed]
43. Ogino, S.; Kawasaki, T.; Kirkner, G.J.; Kraft, P.; Loda, M.; Fuchs, C.S. Evaluation of markers for CpG island methylator phenotype (CIMP) in colorectal cancer by a large population-based sample. *J. Mol. Diagn.* **2007**, *9*, 305–314. [CrossRef] [PubMed]
44. Samowitz, W.S.; Albertsen, H.; Herrick, J.; Levin, T.R.; Sweeney, C.; Murtaugh, M.A.; Wolff, R.K.; Slattery, M.L. Evaluation of a large, population-based sample supports a CpG island methylator phenotype in colon cancer. *Gastroenterology* **2005**, *129*, 837–845. [CrossRef] [PubMed]
45. Gaiani, F.; Marchesi, F.; Negri, F.; Greco, L.; Malesci, A.; de'Angelis, G.L.; Laghi, L. Heterogeneity of Colorectal Cancer Progression: Molecular Gas and Brakes. *Int. J. Mol. Sci.* **2021**, *22*, 5246. [CrossRef] [PubMed]

46. Kambara, T.; Simms, L.A.; Whitehall, V.L.; Spring, K.J.; Wynter, C.V.; Walsh, M.D.; Barker, M.A.; Arnold, S.; McGivern, A.; Matsubara, N.; et al. BRAF mutation is associated with DNA methylation in serrated polyps and cancers of the colorectum. *Gut* **2004**, *53*, 1137–1144. [CrossRef] [PubMed]
47. Nosho, K.; Irahara, N.; Shima, K.; Kure, S.; Kirkner, G.J.; Schernhammer, E.S.; Hazra, A.; Hunter, D.J.; Quackenbush, J.; Spiegelman, D.; et al. Comprehensive biostatistical analysis of CpG island methylator phenotype in colorectal cancer using a large population-based sample. *PLoS ONE* **2008**, *3*, e3698. [CrossRef] [PubMed]
48. Ref Merlo, A.; Herman, J.G.; Mao, L.; Lee, D.J.; Gabrielson, E.; Burger, P.C.; Baylin, S.B.; Sidransky, D. 5' CpG island methylation is associated with transcriptional silencing of the tumour suppressor p16/CDKN2/MTS1 in human cancers. *Nat. Med.* **1995**, *1*, 686–692. [CrossRef] [PubMed]
49. Warthin, A.S. Heredity with reference to carcinoma as shown by the study of the cases examined in the Pathological Laboratory of the University of Michigan, 1895–1912. *Arch. Int. Med.* **1913**, *12*, 546–555. [CrossRef]
50. Boland, C.R.; Lynch, H.T. The history of Lynch syndrome. *Fam. Cancer* **2013**, *12*, 145–157. [CrossRef]
51. Lynch, H.T.; Kimberling, W.; Albano, W.A.; Lynch, J.F.; Biscone, K.; Schuelke, G.S.; Sandberg, A.A.; Lipkin, M.; Deschner, E.E.; Mikol, Y.B.; et al. Hereditary nonpolyposis colorectal cancer (Lynch syndromes I and II). I. Clinical description of resource. *Cancer* **1985**, *56*, 934–938. [CrossRef]
52. Carethers, J.M.; Stoffel, E.M. Lynch syndrome and Lynch syndrome mimics: The growing complex landscape of hereditary colon cancer. *World J. Gastroenterol.* **2015**, *21*, 9253–9261. [CrossRef]
53. Pico, M.D.; Castillejo, A.; Murcia, O.; Giner-Calabuig, M.; Alustiza, M.; Sanchez, A.; Moreira, L.; Pellise, M.; Castells, A.; Carrillo-Palau, M.; et al. Clinical and Pathological Characterization of Lynch-Like Syndrome. *Clin. Gastroenterol. Hepatol.* **2020**, *18*, 368–374. [CrossRef]
54. Rodriguez-Soler, M.; Perez-Carbonell, L.; Guarinos, C.; Zapater, P.; Castillejo, A.; Barbera, V.M.; Juarez, M.; Bessa, X.; Xicola, R.M.; Clofent, J.; et al. Risk of cancer in cases of suspected lynch syndrome without germline mutation. *Gastroenterology* **2013**, *144*, 926.e921–932.e921, quiz e913–e924. [CrossRef] [PubMed]
55. Mensenkamp, A.R.; Vogelaar, I.P.; van Zelst-Stams, W.A.; Goossens, M.; Ouchene, H.; Hendriks-Cornelissen, S.J.; Kwint, M.P.; Hoogerbrugge, N.; Nagtegaal, I.D.; Ligtenberg, M.J. Somatic mutations in MLH1 and MSH2 are a frequent cause of mismatch-repair deficiency in Lynch syndrome-like tumors. *Gastroenterology* **2014**, *146*, 643.e648–646.e648. [CrossRef] [PubMed]
56. Sankila, R.; Aaltonen, L.A.; Järvinen, H.J.; Mecklin, J.P. Better survival rates in patients with MLH1-associated hereditary colorectal cancer. *Gastroenterology* **1996**, *110*, 682–687. [CrossRef]
57. Gryfe, R.; Gallinger, S. Microsatellite instability, mismatch repair deficiency, and colorectal cancer. *Surgery* **2001**, *130*, 17–20. [CrossRef] [PubMed]
58. Dienstmann, R.; Mason, M.J.; Sinicrope, F.A.; Phipps, A.I.; Tejpar, S.; Nesbakken, A.; Danielsen, S.A.; Sveen, A.; Buchanan, D.D.; Clendenning, M.; et al. Prediction of overall survival in stage II and III colon cancer beyond TNM system: A retrospective, pooled biomarker study. *Ann. Oncol.* **2017**, *28*, 1023–1031. [CrossRef]
59. Sargent, D.J.; Shi, Q.; Yothers, G.; Tejpar, S.; Bertagnolli, M.M.; Thibodeau, S.N.; Andre, T.; Labianca, R.; Gallinger, S.; Hamilton, S.R.; et al. Prognostic impact of deficient mismatch repair (dMMR) in 7,803 stage II/III colon cancer (CC) patients (pts): A pooled individual pt data analysis of 17 adjuvant trials in the ACCENT database. *J. Clin. Oncol.* **2014**, *32*, 3507. [CrossRef]
60. Klingbiel, D.; Saridaki, Z.; Roth, A.D.; Bosman, F.T.; Delorenzi, M.; Tejpar, S. Prognosis of stage II and III colon cancer treated with adjuvant 5-fluorouracil or FOLFIRI in relation to microsatellite status: Results of the PETACC–3 trial. *Ann. Oncol.* **2015**, *26*, 126–132. [CrossRef] [PubMed]
61. Wang, B.; Li, F.; Zhou, X.; Ma, Y.; Fu, W. Is microsatellite instability-high really a favorable prognostic factor for advanced colorectal cancer? A meta-analysis. *World J. Surg. Oncol.* **2019**, *17*, 169. [CrossRef]
62. Buckowitz, A.; Knaebel, H.P.; Benner, A.; Blaker, H.; Gebert, J.; Kienle, P.; von Doeberitz, K.M.; Kloor, M. Microsatellite instability in colorectal cancer is associated with local lymphocyte infiltration and low frequency of distant metastases. *Br. J. Cancer* **2005**, *92*, 1746–1753. [CrossRef] [PubMed]
63. Venderbosch, S.; Nagtegaal, I.D.; Maughan, T.S.; Smith, C.G.; Cheadle, J.P.; Fisher, D.; Kaplan, R.; Quirke, P.; Seymour, M.T.; Richman, S.D.; et al. Mismatch repair status and BRAF mutation status in metastatic colorectal cancer patients: A pooled analysis of the CAIRO, CAIRO2, COIN, and FOCUS studies. *Clin. Cancer Res.* **2014**, *20*, 5322–5330. [CrossRef]
64. Laghi, L.; Bianchi, P.; Miranda, E.; Balladore, E.; Pacetti, V.; Grizzi, F.; Allavena, P.; Torri, V.; Repici, A.; Santoro, A.; et al. CD3+ cells at the invasive margin of deeply invading (pT3-T4) colorectal cancer and risk of post-surgical metastasis: A longitudinal study. *Lancet Oncol.* **2009**, *10*, 877–884. [CrossRef]
65. Pagès, F.; Kirilovsky, A.; Mlecnik, B.; Asslaber, M.; Tosolini, M.; Bindea, G.; Galon, J. In situ cytotoxic and memory T cells predict outcome in patients with early stage colorectal cancer. *J. Clin. Oncol.* **2009**, *27*, 5944–5951. [CrossRef] [PubMed]
66. Lin, A.; Zhang, J.; Luo, P. Crosstalk Between the MSI Status and Tumor Microenvironment in Colorectal Cancer. *Front Immunol.* **2020**, *11*, 2039. [CrossRef]
67. Galon, J.; Mlecnik, B.; Bindea, G.; Angell, H.K.; Berger, A.; Lagorce, C.; Pagès, F. Towards the introduction of the 'Immunoscore' in the classification of malignant tumours. *J. Pathol.* **2014**, *232*, 199–209. [CrossRef]
68. Wirta, E.V.; Seppälä, T.; Friman, M.; Väyrynen, J.; Ahtiainen, M.; Kautiainen, H.; Kuopio, T.; Kellokumpu, I.; Mecklin, J.P.; Böhm, J. Immunoscore in mismatch repair-proficient and -deficient colon cancer. *J. Pathol. Clin. Res.* **2017**, *3*, 203–213. [CrossRef] [PubMed]

69. Noepel-Duennebacke, S.; Juette, H.; Schulmann, K.; Graeven, U.; Porschen, R.; Stoehlmacher, J.; Hegewisch-Becker, S.; Raulf, A.; Arnold, D.; Reinacher-Schick, A.; et al. Microsatellite instability (MSI-H) is associated with a high immunoscore but not with PD-L1 expression or increased survival in patients (pts.) with metastatic colorectal cancer (mCRC) treated with oxaliplatin (ox) and fluoropyrimidine (FP) with and without bevacizumab (bev): A pooled analysis of the AIO KRK 0207 and RO91 trials. *J. Cancer Res. Clin. Oncol.* **2021**, *147*, 3063–3072.
70. Ribic, C.M.; Sargent, D.J.; Moore, M.J.; Thibodeau, S.N.; French, A.J.; Goldberg, R.M.; Gallinger, S. Tumor microsatellite-instability status as a predictor of benefit from fluorouracil-based adjuvant chemotherapy for colon cancer. *N. Engl. J. Med.* **2003**, *349*, 247–257. [CrossRef] [PubMed]
71. Sargent, D.J.; Marsoni, S.; Monges, G.; Thibodeau, S.N.; Labianca, R.; Hamilton, S.R.; French, A.J.; Kabat, B.; Foster, N.R.; Torri, V.; et al. Defective mismatch repair as a predictive marker for lack of efficacy of fluorouracil-based adjuvant therapy in colon cancer. *J. Clin. Oncol.* **2010**, *28*, 3219–3226. [CrossRef] [PubMed]
72. Sinicrope, F.A.; Foster, N.R.; Thibodeau, S.N.; Marsoni, S.; Monges, G.; Labianca, R.; Kim, G.P.; Yothers, G.; Allegra, C.; Moore, M.J.; et al. DNA mismatch repair status and colon cancer recurrence and survival in clinical trials of 5-fluorouracil-based adjuvant therapy. *J. Natl. Cancer Inst.* **2011**, *103*, 863–875. [CrossRef] [PubMed]
73. Hutchins, G.; Southward, K.; Handley, K.; Magill, L.; Beaumont, C.; Stahlschmidt, J.; Richman, S.; Chambers, P.; Seymour, M.; Kerr, D.; et al. Value of mismatch repair, KRAS, and BRAF mutations in predicting recurrence and benefits from chemotherapy in colorectal cancer. *J. Clin. Oncol.* **2011**, *29*, 1261–1270. [CrossRef]
74. Petrelli, F.; Ghidini, M.; Cabiddu, M.; Pezzica, E.; Corti, D.; Turati, L.; Costanzo, A.; Varricchio, A.; Ghidini, A.; Barni, S.; et al. Microsatellite Instability and Survival in Stage II Colorectal Cancer: A Systematic Review and Meta-analysis. *Anticancer Res.* **2019**, *39*, 6431–6441. [CrossRef] [PubMed]
75. Fomiti, A.; Rulli, E.; Pilozzi, E.; Gerardi, C.; Roberto, M.; Legramandi, L.; Falcone, R.; Pacchetti, I.; Marchetti, P.; Floriani, I. Exploring the prognostic role of microsatellite instability in patients with stage II colorectal cancer: A systematic review and meta-analysis. *Clin. Colorectal Cancer* **2017**, *16*, e55–e59.
76. Laghi, L.; Malesci, A. Microsatellite instability and therapeutic consequences in colorectal cancer. *Dig. Dis.* **2012**, *30*, 304–309. [CrossRef] [PubMed]
77. Koopman, M.; Kortman, G.A.; Mekenkamp, L.; Ligtenberg, M.J.; Hoogerbrugge, N.; Antonini, N.F.; Punt, C.J.; van Krieken, J.H. Deficient mismatch repair system in patients with sporadic advanced colorectal cancer. *Br. J. Cancer* **2009**, *100*, 266–273. [CrossRef] [PubMed]
78. Sinicrope, F.A.; Mahoney, M.R.; Smyrk, T.C.; Thibodeau, S.N.; Warren, R.S.; Bertagnolli, M.M.; Nelson, G.D.; Goldberg, R.M.; Sargent, D.J.; Alberts, S.R. Prognostic impact of deficient DNA mismatch repair in patients with stage III colon cancer from a randomized trial of FOLFOX-based adjuvant chemotherapy. *J. Clin. Oncol.* **2013**, *31*, 3664–3672. [CrossRef] [PubMed]
79. Emile, J.F.; Julié, C.; Le Malicot, K.; Lepage, C.; Tabernero, J.; Mini, E.; Budnik, T.M. Prospective validation of a lymphocyte infiltration prognostic test in stage III colon cancer patients treated with adjuvant FOLFOX. *Eur. J. Cancer* **2017**, *82*, 16–24. [CrossRef]
80. Zaanan, A.; Shi, Q.; Taieb, J.; Alberts, S.R.; Meyers, J.P.; Smyrk, T.C.; Julie, C.; Zawadi, A.; Tabernero, J.; Mini, E.; et al. Role of Deficient DNA Mismatch Repair Status in Patients with Stage III Colon Cancer Treated with FOLFOX Adjuvant Chemotherapy: A Pooled Analysis From 2 Randomized Clinical Trials. *JAMA Oncol.* **2018**, *4*, 379–383. [CrossRef] [PubMed]
81. Kucherlapati, M.H.; Lee, K.; Nguyen, A.A.; Clark, A.B.; Hou, H., Jr.; Rosulek, A.; Li, H.; Yang, K.; Fan, K.; Lipkin, M.; et al. An Msh2 conditional knockout mouse for studying intestinal cancer and testing anticancer agents. *Gastroenterology* **2010**, *138*, 993.e1–1002.e1. [CrossRef]
82. Gavin, P.G.; Colangelo, L.H.; Fumagalli, D.; Tanaka, N.; Remillard, M.Y.; Yothers, G.; Kim, C.; Taniyama, Y.; Kim, S.I.; Choi, H.J.; et al. Mutation profiling and microsatellite instability in stage II and III colon cancer: An assessment of their prognostic and oxaliplatin predictive value. *Clin. Cancer Res.* **2012**, *18*, 6531–6541. [CrossRef]
83. Taieb, J.; Le Malicot, K.; Shi, Q.; Penault-Llorca, F.; Bouché, O.; Tabernero, J.; Mini, E.; Goldberg, R.M.; Folprecht, G.; Luc Van Laethem, J.; et al. Prognostic Value of BRAF and KRAS Mutations in MSI and MSS Stage III Colon Cancer. *J. Natl. Cancer Inst.* **2016**, *109*, 272. [CrossRef] [PubMed]
84. Rizvi, N.A.; Hellmann, M.D.; Snyder, A.; Kvistborg, P.; Makarov, V.; Havel, J.J.; Lee, W.; Yuan, J.; Wong, P.; Ho, T.S.; et al. Cancer immunology. Mutational landscape determines sensitivity to PD−1 blockade in non-small cell lung cancer. *Science* **2015**, *348*, 124–128. [CrossRef] [PubMed]
85. Giannakis, M.; Mu, X.J.; Shukla, S.A.; Qian, Z.R.; Cohen, O.; Nishihara, R.; Garraway, L.A. Genomic correlates of immune-cell infiltrates in colorectal carcinoma. *Cell Rep.* **2016**, *15*, 857–865. [CrossRef]
86. Le, D.T.; Durham, J.N.; Smith, K.N.; Wang, H.; Bartlett, B.R.; Aulakh, L.K.; Diaz, L.A. Mismatch repair deficiency predicts response of solid tumors to PD−1 blockade. *Science* **2017**, *357*, 409–413. [CrossRef] [PubMed]
87. Roudko, V.; Bozkus, C.C.; Orfanelli, T.; McClain, C.B.; Carr, C.; O'Donnell, T.; Chakraborty, L.; Samstein, R.; Huang, K.L.; Blank, S.V.; et al. Shared Immunogenic Poly-Epitope Frameshift Mutations in Microsatellite Unstable Tumors. *Cell* **2020**, *183*, 1634–1649.e17. [CrossRef] [PubMed]
88. Llosa, N.J.; Cruise, M.; Tam, A.; Wicks, E.C.; Hechenbleikner, E.M.; Taube, J.M.; Blosser, R.L.; Fan, H.; Wang, H.; Luber, B.S.; et al. The vigorous immune microenvironment of microsatellite instable colon cancer is balanced by multiple counter-inhibitory checkpoints. *Cancer Discov.* **2015**, *5*, 43–51. [CrossRef] [PubMed]

89. Le, D.T.; Uram, J.N.; Wang, H.; Bartlett, B.R.; Kemberling, H.; Eyring, A.D.; Diaz, L.A., Jr. PD−1 blockade in tumors with mismatch-repair deficiency. *N. Engl. J. Med.* **2015**, *372*, 2509–2520. [CrossRef] [PubMed]
90. Overman, M.J.; Lonardi, S.; Wong, K.Y.M.; Lenz, H.J.; Gelsomino, F.; Aglietta, M.; André, T. Durable clinical benefit with nivolumab plus ipilimumab in DNA mismatch repair-deficient/microsatellite instability-high metastatic colorectal cancer. *J. Clin. Oncol.* **2018**, *36*, 773–779. [CrossRef] [PubMed]
91. Ursem, C.; Atreya, C.E.; Van Loon, K. Emerging treatment options for BRAF-mutant colorectal cancer. *Gastrointest. Cancer* **2018**, *8*, 13–23. [CrossRef]
92. The Cancer Genome Atlas Network. Comprehensive molecular characterization of human colon and rectal cancer. *Nature* **2012**, *487*, 330–337. [CrossRef] [PubMed]
93. Tran, B.; Kopetz, S.; Tie, J.; Gibbs, P.; Jiang, Z.Q.; Lieu, C.H.; Desai, J. Impact of BRAF mutation and microsatellite instability on the pattern of metastatic spread and prognosis in metastatic colorectal cancer. *Cancer* **2011**, *117*, 4623–4632. [CrossRef]
94. Hyman, D.M.; Puzanov, I.; Subbiah, V.; Faris, J.E.; Chau, I.; Blay, J.Y.; Baselga, J. Vemurafenib in multiple nonmelanoma cancers with BRAF V600 mutations. *N. Engl. J. Med.* **2015**, *373*, 726–736. [CrossRef]
95. Corcoran, R.B.; Atreya, C.E.; Falchook, G.S.; Kwak, E.L.; Ryan, D.P.; Bendell, J.C.; Hamid, O.; Messersmith, W.A.; Daud, A.; Kurzrock, R.; et al. Combined BRAF and MEK Inhibition with Dabrafenib and Trametinib in BRAF V600-Mutant Colorectal Cancer. *J. Clin. Oncol.* **2015**, *33*, 4023–4031. [CrossRef]
96. Corcoran, R.B.; André, T.; Atreya, C.E.; Schellens, J.H.M.; Yoshino, T.; Bendell, J.C.; Hollebecque, A.; McRee, A.J.; Siena, S.; Middleton, G.; et al. Combined BRAF, EGFR, and MEK Inhibition in Patients with BRAFV600E-Mutant Colorectal Cancer. *Cancer Discov.* **2018**, *8*, 428–443. [CrossRef] [PubMed]
97. Tahara, T.; Yamamoto, E.; Suzuki, H.; Maruyama, R.; Chung, W.; Garriga, J.; Issa, J.P.J. Fusobacterium in colonic flora and molecular features of colorectal carcinoma. *Cancer Res.* **2014**, *74*, 1311–1318. [CrossRef]
98. Mima, K.; Cao, Y.; Chan, A.T.; Qian, Z.R.; Nowak, J.A.; Masugi, Y.; Ogino, S. Fusobacterium nucleatum in colorectal carcinoma tissue according to tumor location. *Gut* **2016**, *65*, 1973–1980. [CrossRef] [PubMed]
99. Hamada, T.; Zhang, X.; Mima, K.; Bullman, S.; Sukawa, Y.; Nowak, J.A.; Kosumi, K.; Masugi, Y.; Twombly, T.S.; Cao, Y.; et al. Fusobacterium nucleatum in Colorectal Cancer Relates to Immune Response Differentially by Tumor Microsatellite Instability Status. *Cancer Immunol. Res.* **2018**, *6*, 1327–1336. [CrossRef] [PubMed]
100. Compton, C.C.; Sullivan, D.C.; Byrd, D.R.; Greene, F.L.; Gershenwald, J.E.; Hess, K.R.; Gaspar, L.E.; Washington, M.K.; Schilsky, R.L.; Edge, S. *AJCC Cancer Staging Manual*, 8th ed.; Amin, M.B., Edge, S.B., Greene, F.L., Byrd, D.R., Brookland, R.K., Washington, M.K., Gershenwald, J.E., Compton, C.C., Hess, K.R., Sullivan, D.C., Jessup, J.M., Brierley, J.D., Gaspar, L.E., Schilsky, R.L., Balch, C.M., Winchester, D.P., Asare, E.A., Madera, M., Gress, D.M., Meyer, L.R., Eds.; Springer International Publishing: New York, NY, USA, 2017.

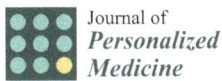

Article

LAG-3 Expression Predicts Outcome in Stage II Colon Cancer

Gaëlle Rhyner Agocs [1,2], Naziheh Assarzadegan [3,4], Richard Kirsch [3], Heather Dawson [5], José A. Galván [5], Alessandro Lugli [5], Inti Zlobec [5] and Martin D. Berger [1,*]

1. Department of Medical Oncology, Inselspital, Bern University Hospital, University of Bern, 3010 Bern, Switzerland; Gaelle.Rhyner@h-fr.ch
2. Department of Medical Oncology, HFR Fribourg Hospital, 1708 Fribourg, Switzerland
3. Division of Pathology and Lab Medicine, University of Toronto, Toronto, ON M5G 1X5, Canada; nassarz1@jhmi.edu (N.A.); Richard.Kirsch@sinaihealth.ca (R.K.)
4. Department of Pathology, The Johns Hopkins University School of Medicine, Baltimore, MD 21212, USA
5. Institute of Pathology, University of Bern, 3008 Bern, Switzerland; heather.dawson@pathology.unibe.ch (H.D.); jose.galvan@pathology.unibe.ch (J.A.G.); alessandro.lugli@pathology.unibe.ch (A.L.); inti.zlobec@pathology.unibe.ch (I.Z.)
* Correspondence: martin.berger@insel.ch

Citation: Rhyner Agocs, G.; Assarzadegan, N.; Kirsch, R.; Dawson, H.; Galván, J.A.; Lugli, A.; Zlobec, I.; Berger, M.D. LAG-3 Expression Predicts Outcome in Stage II Colon Cancer. *J. Pers. Med.* **2021**, *11*, 749. https://doi.org/10.3390/jpm11080749

Academic Editors: Enrico Mini and Stefania Nobili

Received: 16 July 2021
Accepted: 20 July 2021
Published: 30 July 2021

Publisher's Note: MDPI stays neutral with regard to jurisdictional claims in published maps and institutional affiliations.

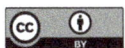

Copyright: © 2021 by the authors. Licensee MDPI, Basel, Switzerland. This article is an open access article distributed under the terms and conditions of the Creative Commons Attribution (CC BY) license (https://creativecommons.org/licenses/by/4.0/).

Abstract: Introduction: LAG-3 is an inhibitory immune checkpoint molecule that suppresses T cell activation and inflammatory cytokine secretion. T cell density in the tumor microenvironment of colon cancer plays an important role in the host's immunosurveillance. We therefore hypothesized that LAG-3 expression on tumor-infiltrating lymphocytes (TILs) predicts outcome in patients with stage II colon cancer. Patients and Methods: Immunohistochemical staining for LAG-3 was performed on tissue microarrays (TMAs) of formalin-fixed paraffin-embedded tissue from 142 stage II colon cancer patients. LAG-3 expression was assessed in TILs within both the tumor front and tumor center and scored as either positive or negative. The primary endpoint was disease-free survival (DFS). Results: In patients diagnosed with stage II colon cancer, the presence of LAG-3 expression on TILs was significantly associated with better 5-year DFS (HR 0.34, 95% CI 0.14–0.80, p = 0.009). The effect on DFS was mainly due to LAG-3-positive TILs in the tumor front (HR 0.33, 95% CI 0.13–0.82, p = 0.012). Conclusion: Assessment of LAG-3 might help to predict outcomes in patients with stage II colon cancer and potentially identify those patients who might benefit from adjuvant chemotherapy. Therefore, LAG-3 may serve as a prognostic biomarker in stage II colon cancer.

Keywords: biomarker; LAG-3; immune checkpoint; colon cancer; survival

1. Introduction

Colon cancer is a major cause of cancer-associated death worldwide and its global incidence is continuously increasing [1,2]. The prognosis of patients with colon cancer is mainly dependent on the stage according to the TNM classification system [3]. While patients diagnosed with stage I colon cancer have an excellent outcome, those with stage IV disease have a low chance of cure and a significantly worse survival [4,5]. Interestingly, some patients with stage II colon cancer, especially the ones with a pT4b tumor (stage IIC), have a worse outcome compared with those with a pT1 or pT2 N+ tumor (stage IIIA and IIIB). In fact, one might assume that a node-positive disease indicates a more aggressive tumor biology translating into a poorer clinical outcome [4]. According to current guidelines, adjuvant chemotherapy is indicated for stage III colon cancer and for stage II disease with additional clinicopathological risk factors [6]. Despite curative surgery and adjuvant chemotherapy, relapses occur and pose significant challenges for our health care system. However, some patients will not benefit from adjuvant chemotherapy because they have already been cured by surgery alone [7]. Therefore, new prognostic and predictive biomarkers have to be developed to define subgroups of patients, especially those with low- or standard risk stage II cancer who have a high chance of relapse and may derive the most benefit from chemotherapy [8].

Recently, substantial progress has been made in understanding the role of immune cell infiltration in colon cancer, which has led to the development of the Immunoscore in stage I–III colon cancer, based on the quantification of CD3+ and CD8+ lymphocytes in the tumor and its invasive margin [9]. Remarkably, this scoring system predicts disease-free and overall survival even more precisely than the TNM classification and might therefore guide our treatment decisions in the future [9]. Moreover, the identification of immune-related biomarkers on tumor-infiltrating lymphocytes (TILs) might help to predict prognosis and direct clinical decisions. Recent trials demonstrated that the presence of immune-related biomarkers such as PD-1/PD-L1 on tumor-infiltrating cells might serve as prognostic biomarkers in colorectal cancer [8,10]. The lymphocyte-activation gene 3 (LAG-3 or CD223) is another inhibitory immune-related molecule that is expressed on T cells, especially on activated CD8+ and CD4+ T cells, but also on B cells and dendritic cells, which may act in synergy with the PD-1/PD-L1 pathway [11,12]. LAG-3 mainly binds to the major histocompatibility complex II (MHC II), and thus prevents the interaction of the MHC II with the T cell receptor (TCR) on CD4+ T cells, resulting in decreased CD4+ activity. Another ligand of LAG-3 is Galectin-3, which is mainly expressed on epithelial and immune cells and preferentially binds to LAG-3 on CD8 cells [13]. The protein liver sinusoidal endothelial cell lectin (LSECtin) is a further potential ligand that binds to LAG-3 [14,15]. Upregulation of LAG-3 on immune cells downregulates T cell expansion and cytokine secretion, and thus contributes to an immunosuppressive microenvironment [16,17].

Given the growing interest in the role of LAG-3 in cancer, we sought to evaluate the presence of LAG-3 on tumor-infiltrating lymphocytes (TILs) in the tumor center and tumor front and to assess its impact on outcomes in stage II colon cancer.

2. Patients and Methods

2.1. Patient Cohort

Between 1992 and 2010, patients at the Mount Sinai University Hospital in Toronto, Canada with curatively resected stage II colon cancer in which archival material was available were consecutively included in this retrospective study. Patients with rectal cancers were excluded from our analysis.

A histopathological review was performed according to the 6th edition of the TNM classification system. Clinical data were obtained from patient records. The baseline characteristics comprised age at diagnosis, gender, tumor location, pT stage, tumor grade and lymphatic and venous vessel invasion. In addition, tumor budding, considered as a supplementary prognostic factor, was scored according to the International Tumor Budding Consensus Conference 2016 [18]. Moreover, the mismatch repair (MMR) status was determined by immunohistochemistry. The study was approved by the research ethics board of the Mount Sinai Hospital (nr 13-0136).

2.2. Next-Generation Tissue Microarray (ngTMA®) Construction

H&E-stained (hematoxylin and eosin-stained) whole slides of each case were digitized using a slide scanner (3DHistech, P250, Hungary). Each scan was annotated twice using a 0.6 mm tool in four different regions of interest: tumor center (encompassing mostly tumor epithelium), tumor front (targeting 50% tumor and 50% stromal areas at the invasion front), and tumor stroma (including largely stromal areas at the invasion front with only little, if any tumor). This produced 11 ngTMA® blocks with six cores per tumor.

2.3. Immunohistochemistry

2.5 µm ngTMA® sections were mounted onto glass slides, dried and baked at 60 °C for 30 min prior to use. All immunostainings were performed by automated staining using Bond RX (Leica Biosystems, Muttenz, Switzerland). All slides were dewaxed in Bond dewax solution (product code AR9222, Leica Biosystems). Heat-induced epitope retrieval at pH 9 in Tris buffer base (code AR9640, Leica Biosystems) followed for 30 min at 95 °C. LAG-3 rabbit monoclonal antibody (Cell Signaling, clone D2G4O Ref 15372) was diluted 1:200 and incubated for 30 min at room temperature. Then, the samples underwent incubation with HRP (Horseradish Peroxidase)-polymer for 15 min and were subsequently visualized using 3,3-Diaminobenzidine (DAB) as brown chromogen (Bond polymer refine detection, Leica Biosystems, Ref DS9800) for 10 min. Finally, the samples were counterstained with hematoxylin, dehydrated and mounted with Tissue-Tek® Glas™ Mounting Media (Sakura). Slides were scanned and photographed using Pannoramic 250 (3DHistech). The immunostainings for the mismatch repair proteins were performed using the VENTANA MMR IHC Panel and the VENTANA BenchMark automated staining system (Roche Diagnostics, Mannheim, Germany) according to the manufacturer's instructions. The following antibodies were used: anti-MLH1 (mouse, clone M1, Roche Diagnostics, Ref 8504946001), anti-MSH2 (mouse, clone G219, Roche Diagnostics, Ref 8504946001), anti-MSH6 (rabbit, clone SP93, Roche Diagnostics, Ref 8504946001) and anti-PMS2 (mouse A16-4, Roche Diagnostics, Ref 8504946001).

2.4. Evaluation of Immunohistochemistry

All TMA cores for each individual case were evaluated for the presence or absence of LAG-3 immunohistochemical staining (G.R). Consistent with Sobottka et al., LAG-3 expression on TILs within both the tumor front and tumor center was dichotomously scored as either positive or negative [19]. Representative images are outlined in Figure 1A–D. LAG-3 positivity on TILs was defined as membranous staining of any intensity regardless of the number of LAG-3 positive immune cells (≥ 1), whereas the absence of any staining was determined as LAG-3 negative. We reported the scores for LAG-3 positive TILs as absolute numbers and used the maximum score of all analyzed tissue cores from each patient. The tumor front was defined as the area where the most advancing cancer cells reached the edge of the tumor. In a control set of normal, non-neoplastic colon tissues, no LAG-3 positivity could be observed. Mismatch repair deficiency (dMMR) was defined as the loss of nuclear expression of at least one of the four MMR proteins (MLH1, MSH2, MSH6 and PMS2) in the tumor cells in the presence of an internal positive control such as lymphocytes, normal epithelium or fibroblasts in the close vicinity of the tumor. Focal weak and dotted nuclear staining were considered negative. Retained nuclear expression of all MMR proteins was determined as mismatch repair proficiency (pMMR) [20].

2.5. Statistical Analysis

Correlations between LAG-3 expression in TILs within the tumor center/front and categorical variables were tested using the chi-square test. Continuous or ordinal variables were analyzed with the Kruskal-Wallis or Wilcoxon rank sum test. Disease-free survival (DFS) analysis was performed with Kaplan-Meier survival curves and log-rank test. Hazard ratios and 95% confidence intervals (CIs) were used to determine the effect of each variable on outcome, using Cox regression analysis. DFS was calculated from the time of surgery to local or distant recurrence or death. A p-value < 0.05 was considered statistically significant. Statistical analysis was carried out by SPSS version 26 (United States).

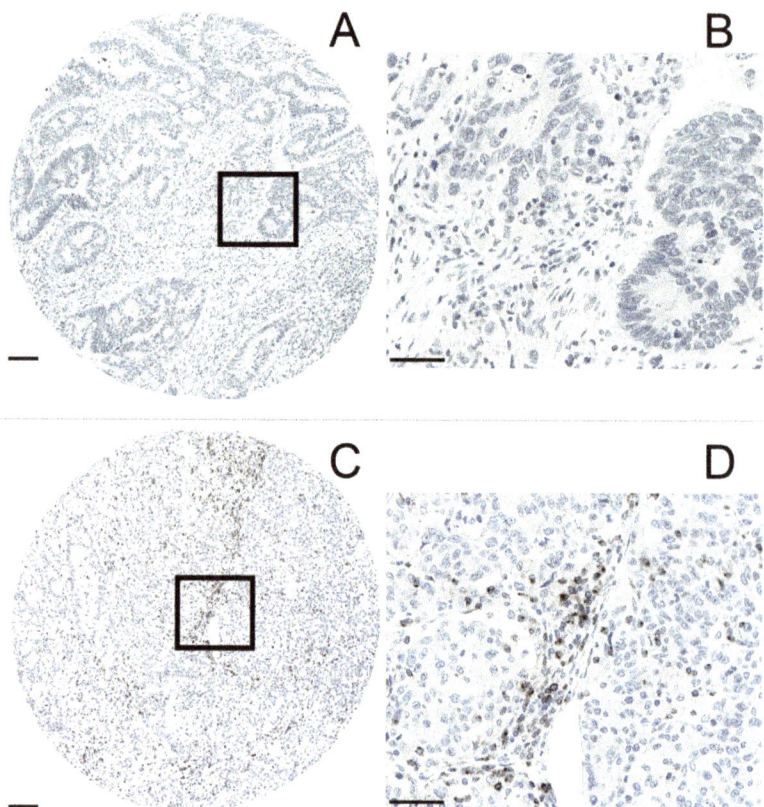

Figure 1. (**A,B**): Absence of immunohistochemical staining for LAG-3 on TILs (magnification: A 5× and B 40×). (**C,D**): TILs expressing LAG-3 (magnification C 5× and D 40×). Scale bar (**A,C**): 100 μm. Scale bar (**B,D**): 50 μm. All images (**A–D**) represent the tumor center.

3. Results

3.1. Patients Characteristics

Our study population comprised 142 patients with curatively resected stage II colon cancer. The median age of the patients was 70 years (range, 24–98 years). 42.2% (n = 60) of the patients were female and 57.8% (n = 82) male. 85.8% (n = 121) of the study cohort had a pT3 tumor, whereas 14.2% (n = 20) of the patients presented with a pT4 tumor. 91% of the tumors (n = 122) were well (G1) or moderately (G2) differentiated and 9% (n = 12) presented with a G3 grading. 87.4% (n = 118) of the tumor specimens displayed no extramural venous invasion (V0), while vascular invasion could be observed in 12.6% (n = 17). There was a slight predominance of left- as compared to right-sided tumors (52.5%, n = 73 versus 47.5%, n = 66). In total, 124 patients (87.3%) had more than 12 lymph nodes examined, whereas the lymph node yield was less than 12 in 12.7% of the patients (n = 18). From 134 evaluable tumor tissue samples, 75.4% (n = 101) were MMR-proficient, whereas 24.6% (n = 33) were MMR-deficient (Supplementary Table S1). The median tumor budding count was 10 (0–74 buds). The 5-year DFS rate of the cohort was 85%.

3.2. LAG-3 Expression on TILs and Its Correlation with Clinicopathological Characteristics

69% (n = 98) of all patients exhibited LAG-3 expression on tumor-infiltrating lymphocytes.

No significant correlation could be observed between LAG-3 expression on TILs and age, gender, pT stage, grade, vascular invasion, tumor location or tumor budding.

Interestingly, the percentage of MMR-deficient colon cancers was higher if LAG-3 positive TILs were present in the tumor front or center. Conversely, a lower ratio of MMR-deficient colon cancers was observed in the absence of LAG-3 positive TILs ($p = 0.034$). Additionally, LAG-3 expression on TILs in the tumor center was associated with better differentiation (grade 1, $p = 0.021$) (Tables 1 and 2).

3.3. LAG-3 Expression on TILs and Its Association with DFS

The presence of LAG-3 expression on TILs either in the tumor front or tumor center was associated with better DFS (5-year DFS 89.9% (LAG-3 positive TILs) versus 74.7% (LAG-3 negative TILs), HR 0.34, 95% CI 0.14–0.80, $p = 0.009$; Figure 2A). Further analysis demonstrated that the favorable association of LAG-3 positive TILs with DFS was restricted to those that were localized at the tumor front (5-year DFS 91.2% versus 75.2%, HR 0.33, 95% CI 0.13–0.82, $p = 0.012$; Figure 2B). Although statistically not significant, there was a trend towards a longer DFS among LAG-3 positive versus LAG-3 negative TILs in the tumor center (5-year DFS 91.3% versus 81.1%, HR 0.42, 95% CI 0.41–1.24, $p = 0.106$; Figure 2C).

Table 1. Association of LAG-3 (combined tumor front and center) with clinicopathological features on the stage II colon cancer cohort.

Feature		Combined		p-Value
		Front and Center negative	Front or Center positive	
Age, years ($n = 141$)	Mean ± SD	69.5 ± 13.8	67.5 ± 15.7	0.493
Gender ($n = 142$)	Male	24 (52.2)	58 (60.4)	0.352
	Female	22 (47.8)	38 (39.6)	
pT ($n = 141$)	pT3	40 (88.9)	81 (84.4)	0.474
	pT4	5 (11.1)	15 (15.6)	
Tumor grade ($n = 134$)	G1/G2	43 (97.8)	79 (87.8)	0.058
	G3	1 (2.2)	11 (12.2)	
EMVI ($n = 135$)	V0	37 (88.1)	81 (87.1)	0.871
	V1	5 (11.9)	12 (12.9)	
Tumor location ($n = 139$)	Left	26 (59.1)	47 (49.5)	0.291
	Right	18 (40.9)	48 (50.5)	
Tumor budding (ITBCC) ($n = 142$)	Mean ± SD	11.1 ± 11.4	11.9 ± 10.8	0.408
MMR status ($n = 134$)	Proficient	35 (87.5)	66 (70.2)	**0.034**
	Deficient	5 (12.5)	28 (29.8)	

Data are presented as n (%), unless otherwise stated. Abbreviations: SD = standard deviation; pT = pathological T stage (TNM classification system); EMVI = extramural vascular invasion; ITBCC = International Tumor Budding Consensus Conference. Bold indicates statistical significant p-values

The favorable association of LAG-3 expression on TILs either in the tumor front or tumor center with the outcome remained significant, even when we considered only MMR-proficient colon cancers (5-year DFS 90.2% versus 67.9%, HR 0.30, 95% CI 0.11–0.83, $p = 0.014$; Figure 3A). Again, the favorable correlation between LAG-3 positive TILs and outcome among MMR-proficient tumors was limited to those localized at the tumor front (Figure 3B), whereas no association with outcome could be observed among LAG-3 positive versus LAG-3 negative TILs in the tumor center (5-year DFS 90.6% versus 75.7%, HR 0.35, 95% CI 0.12–0.99, $p = 0.039$ and 90.4% versus 80.6%, HR 0.44, 95% CI 0.13–1.56, $p = 0.192$, respectively; Figure 3C).

Due to the low number of events in our cohort of stage II colon cancer, we were not able to conduct a multivariate analysis. However, after adjustment for the pT stage in a bivariate analysis, the favorable effect of LAG-3 expression on DFS remained significant (HR 0.35, 95% CI 0.15–0.83, $p = 0.017$).

Table 2. Association of LAG-3 (front/tumor center) with clinicopathological features on the stage II colon cancer cohort.

Feature		Front			Center		
		Negative	Positive	*p*-value	Negative	Positive	*p*-value
Age, years (*n* = 141)	Mean ± SD	69.8 ± 13.9	67.1 ± 14.6	0.316	68.4 ± 14.0	67.7 ± 14.9	0.784
Gender (*n* = 142)	Male	31 (54.4)	51 (60.0)	0.507	52 (56.5)	28 (58.3)	0.837
	Female	26 (45.6)	34 (40.0)		40 (43.5)	20 (41.7)	
pT (*n* = 141)	pT3	48 (85.7)	73 (85.9)	0.978	78 (85.7)	41 (85.4)	0.962
	pT4	8 (14.3)	12 (14.1)		13 (4.3)	7 (14.6)	
Tumor grade (*n* = 134)	G1/G2	52 (96.3)	70 (87.5)	0.08	86 (95.6)	36 (83.7)	**0.021**
	G3	2 (3.7)	10 (12.5)		4 (4.4)	7 (16.3)	
EMVI (*n* = 135)	V0	46 (88.5)	72 (86.8)	1.0	75 (86.2)	42 (91.3)	0.39
	V1	6 (11.5)	11 (13.3)		12 (13.8)	4 (8.7)	
Tumor location (*n* = 139)	Left	33 (60.0)	40 (47.6)	0.168	51 (57.3)	21 (43.8)	0.123
	Right	22 (40.0)	44 (52.4)		38 (42.7)	27 (56.3)	
Tumor budding (ITBCC) (*n* = 142)	Mean ± SD	11.2 ± 11.6	11.9 ± 10.5	0.227	12.5 ± 11.7	10.0 ± 9.3	0.142
MMR status (*n* = 134)	Proficient	45 (86.5)	56 (68.3)	**0.017**	66 (75.0)	35 (76.1)	0.89
	Deficient	7 (13.5)	26 (31.7)		22 (25.0)	11 (23.9)	

Data are presented as *n* (%), unless otherwise stated. SD = standard deviation; pT = pathological T stage (TNM classification system); EMVI = extramural vascular invasion; ITBCC = International Tumor Budding Consensus Conference. Bold indicates statistical significant *p*-values.

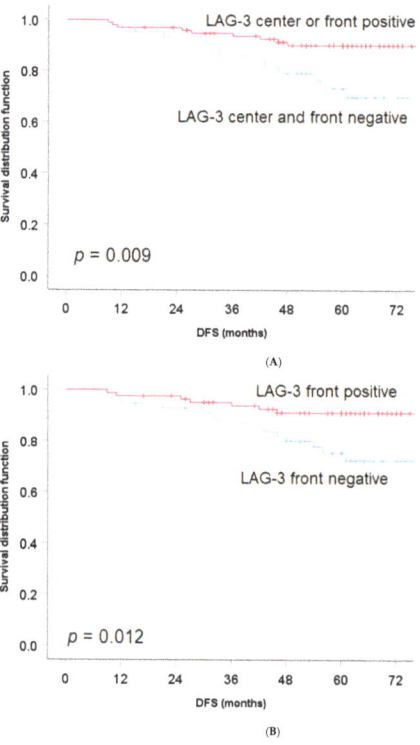

Figure 2. *Cont.*

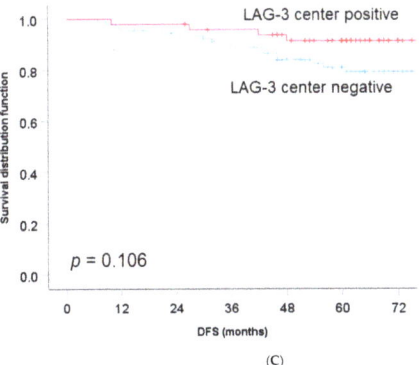

(C)

Figure 2. (**A**): The impact of LAG-3 expression on TILs on DFS in patients with stage II colon cancer (tumor center and tumor front). (**B**): LAG-3 expression on TILs at tumor front and its effect on DFS in stage II colon cancer. (**C**): LAG-3 expression on TILs in the tumor center and its impact on DFS in stage II colon cancer.

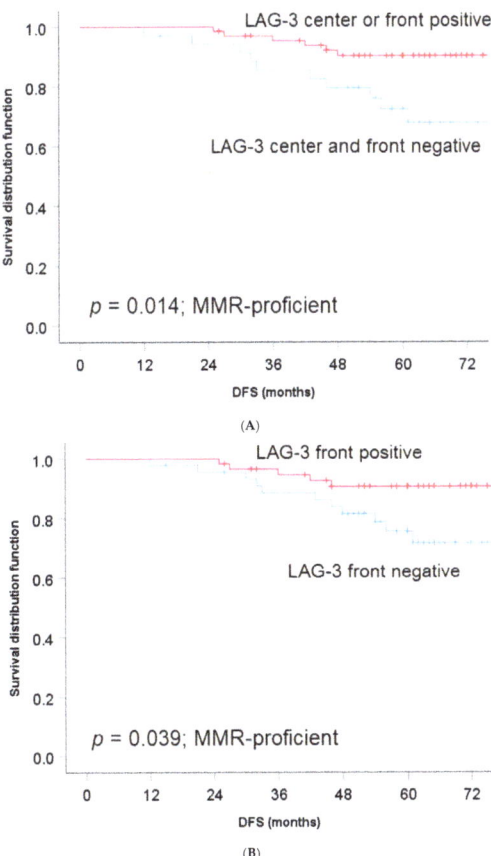

(A)

(B)

Figure 3. *Cont.*

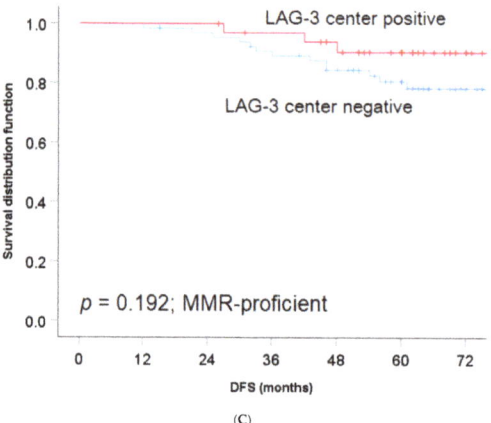

Figure 3. (**A**): The impact of LAG-3 expression on TILs on DFS in patients with stage II MMR-proficient colon cancer (tumor center and tumor front). (**B**): LAG-3 expression on TILs at tumor front and its effect on DFS in stage II MMR-proficient colon cancer. (**C**): LAG-3 expression on TILs in the tumor center and its impact on DFS in stage II MMR-proficient colon cancer.

4. Discussion

To the best of our knowledge, this is the first study evaluating the impact of LAG-3 expression on disease-free survival in stage II colon cancer patients. We demonstrated that LAG-3 expression on TILs was associated with a favorable DFS, especially when LAG-3 positive TILs were identified at the tumor front.

Our results are consistent with previous findings from other studies. Lee et al. found that patients with stage I–III MMR-deficient colon cancer exhibiting LAG-3 positive TILs had a longer DFS compared to those whose MSI tumors did not contain LAG-3 positive TILs [21]. However, in contrast to our study, Lee et al. included only patients with MSI-high tumors ranging from stage I to stage III, whereas our cohort comprised a homogenous series of patients with stage II colon cancer. Additionally, we did not restrict our analysis to patients with MSI stage II colon cancers alone, but also included patients with MSS tumors, representing the majority of stage II cancer patients.

This is particularly important, as we know from previous studies that not only MSI but also MSS tumors may be enriched by immune infiltrates, representing an immunogenic tumor microenvironment (TME) [22]. In a recently published landmark study comprising tumor tissue samples from 2681 patients with stage I–III colon cancer, Pagès et al. could demonstrate that the numbers of CD3+ and cytotoxic CD8+ T cells in the tumor directly correlated with time to recurrence in both the training and validation cohorts, independent of MSI, T and N stages and other clinicopathological factors. A high Immunoscore was not only associated with a longer time to recurrence (TTR) but also translated into better disease-free survival (DFS) and overall survival (OS). Remarkably, patients with a MSI tumor and a high Immunoscore had a similar outcome compared with those who presented with a MSS tumor and a high Immunoscore. Conversely, patients with MSI tumors and a low Immunoscore exhibited a shorter DFS than those with MSS tumors and a high Immunoscore. In the subgroup of stage II colon cancer patients, these associations remained significant [9].

Thus, further characterization of the TME in both MSI and MSS colon cancers is of utmost importance to gain insight into the complex interplay between immune stimulatory and inhibitory effects within the TME to improve our treatment strategies and to better identify patients who benefit most from systemic treatment.

Similarly, Zhang et al. could demonstrate that LAG-3 expression in a mixed cohort of patients with esophageal squamous cell carcinoma encompassing all stages (I–IV) was associated with improved survival, whereas the favorable effect of high versus low LAG-3 expression on outcome was restricted to stage I–II cancers [23]. In an unselected cohort of patients with stage I –IIIB non-small cell lung cancer, including mainly squamous cell carcinoma and adenocarcinoma but also other histological types such as adenosquamous and large cell carcinoma, LAG-3 expression on TILs was correlated with improved survival [24].

Likewise, another study demonstrated that the presence of LAG-3 positive intraepithelial TILs was associated with a longer disease-specific survival among estrogen receptor-negative breast cancer patients [25].

At first glance, it may not seem obvious that the expression of an inhibitory immune-checkpoint molecule such as LAG-3 correlates with a favorable outcome in various solid tumors. Rather, one may assume that the presence of LAG-3 results in increased inhibition of both T cell activation and proliferation and thus contributes to an immune-suppressive tumor microenvironment facilitating tumor growth and metastasis. However, the increased expression of LAG-3 on TILs may not be seen as an independent and 'isolated' immune-inhibiting effect but rather be interpreted as an indicator of an enhanced inflammatory immune response, where TILs are stimulated to exert their antitumor response.

Contrary to our results, Chen et al. reported that patients with stage I–IV colorectal cancer exhibiting a high percentage of LAG-3+ cells in the tumor tissue had a shorter survival compared with those with a low percentage of LAG-3+ cells [26]. However, there are several reasons for these opposite findings. First, the study cohort of Chen et al. comprised 108 patients with a mixture of stage I to stage IV colon and rectal cancers, whereas our cohort consisted of stage II patients with colon cancer alone. Interestingly, Chen et al. found that the percentage of LAG-3+ cells in tumor tissues was significantly higher in stage III and IV colorectal cancers compared to that observed in stage I and II cancers. Given that two-thirds of the patients included in the cohort of Chen et al. had stage III and IV colorectal cancers, it might not be surprising that high versus low LAG-3+ expression in the mixed stage I–IV cohort was associated with shorter survival. Additionally, they could demonstrate that a higher percentage of LAG-3+ cells was associated with poor differentiation, lymph node metastasis and invasion [26], whereas no correlation of LAG-3 expression with any of the clinicopathological characteristics such as tumor grade, vascular invasion or tumor budding could be observed in our study cohort of stage II colon cancer. However, we could demonstrate an association between LAG-3 counts and MMR status. Whereas high LAG-3 expression at the tumor front correlated with microsatellite instability (MSI), this association could not be observed in the tumor center. Second, there is no established scoring method for LAG-3. While Chen et al. divided the cohort into tumors with high and low LAG-3-expressing cells [26], we classified our study cohort according to Sobottka et al. [19], into those tumors exhibiting either LAG+ or LAG- TILs at the tumor front or center. Third, there is a significant diversity of antibodies used for immunohistochemistry across several studies. While we used a rabbit monoclonal antibody (Cell Signaling, clone D2G4O Ref 15372), Chen et al. utilized a different LAG-3 antibody from Abcam (Cambridge, MA, USA) without providing any further information [26].

All these different points mentioned above may partly explain the contradictory findings among our studies. Therefore, it is crucial to develop a standard protocol regarding LAG-3 scoring enabling us to better interpret findings from various studies. Saleh et al. could demonstrate that LAG-3 mRNA expression levels in tumor tissues versus paired normal tissues of colorectal cancer patients were approximately similar [27]. Additionally, Toor et al. could demonstrate in a small and mixed cohort of stage I–IV colorectal cancer patients using a flow cytometry assay that LAG-3 expression on peripheral mononuclear leukocytes was significantly lower compared to the levels observed on both tumor-infiltrating lymphocytes (TILs) and lymphocytes from adjacent normal colon tissue (NILs). Again, no significant difference in LAG-3 expression could be detected between TILs and NILs [28].

With the introduction of immune checkpoint therapies such as PD1 and PD-L1 inhibitors, the prognosis of cancer patients with various malignancies such as melanoma [29], non-small cell lung cancer [30], renal carcinoma [31], urothelial carcinoma [32], head and neck carcinoma [33] and Hodgkin lymphoma has significantly improved [34]. Currently, there are several clinical trials evaluating the effect of LAG-3 inhibitors in different tumor types [35,36]. Therefore, both the diagnostic and therapeutic value of LAG-3 might be evolving in the near future. Whereas immune checkpoint therapy is associated with improved tumor control and longer survival in patients with MSI metastatic colorectal cancer (mCRC), and thus represents the standard of care treatment [37,38], its effect on outcome in patients with microsatellite stable (MSS) mCRC, who represent 95% of all patients with mCRC, is so far disappointing [39]. Additionally, the role of immune checkpoint therapy as part of the adjuvant treatment strategy in both MSS and MSI stage II and stage III still remains elusive, with several studies ongoing [40,41].

The limitations of this study are its monocentric retrospective design, the small sample size and the lack of an independent clinical validation cohort. Moreover, we restricted our analysis to the immunohistochemical assessment of LAG-3 without using further assays such as in situ hybridization or assessment of ELISA serum LAG-3 concentrations. The latter could not be done due to the lack of blood samples. Additionally, the lack of a consensus guideline regarding immunohistochemical LAG-3 scoring makes it challenging to draw any cross-comparisons between studies. However, our strengths are that we restricted our analysis to a well-defined homogenous cohort of patients with stage II colon cancer. In accordance with Sobottka et al., we performed a binary scoring algorithm for LAG-3 expression. By using a dichotomous scoring method rather than a quantitative scoring method with different thresholds, we may minimize the interobserver variability, increase the reproducibility and facilitate further clinical validation studies in other patient cohorts. Given the lack of a general scoring guideline, this simple binary assessment of LAG-3 allows for efficient, cost-effective and easily reproducible scoring that might be implemented in the diagnostic algorithm of stage II colon cancer, enabling clinicians to decide whether a patient should undergo adjuvant chemotherapy.

5. Conclusions

In conclusion, we were able to demonstrate that LAG-3 expression on TILs at the tumor front of stage II colon cancers was associated with better outcomes in both the overall stage II cohort and within the subgroup of stage II MSS tumors. Therefore, LAG-3 might serve as a potential prognostic biomarker. However, further studies are needed to explore whether the assessment of LAG-3 in stage II colon cancer may help us to identify those patients who derive the most benefit from adjuvant chemotherapy.

Supplementary Materials: The following are available online at https://www.mdpi.com/article/10.3390/jpm11080749/s1, Table S1: Baseline characteristics.

Author Contributions: Conceptualization, M.D.B.; methodology, G.R.A., J.A.G., I.Z. and M.D.B.; software, I.Z., J.A.G.; formal analysis, I.Z.; investigation, G.R.A., N.A., R.K., H.D., J.A.G., A.L., I.Z. and M.D.B.; resources, N.A., R.K., H.D., A.L., I.Z. and M.D.B.; data curation, I.Z.; writing–original draft preparation, G.R.A., J.A.G., I.Z. and M.D.B.; writing–review and editing, G.R.A., N.A., R.K., H.D., J.A.G., A.L., I.Z. and M.D.B.; visualization, G.R.A., J.A.G., I.Z.; supervision, M.D.B.; project administration, G.R.A., N.A., R.K., A.L., I.Z., M.D.B.; funding acquisition, M.D.B. All authors have read and agreed to the published version of the manuscript.

Funding: MDB received a grant from the "Bernese Foundation of Clinical Cancer Research".

Institutional Review Board Statement: The study was approved by the research ethics board of the Mount Sinai Hospital (nr 13-0136).

Informed Consent Statement: Since this was a retrospective tissue study, no informed consent was required from the research ethics board.

Data Availability Statement: The data presented in this study are available from the corresponding author upon reasonable request.

Conflicts of Interest: The authors declare no conflict of interest.

References

1. Bray, F.; Me, J.F.; Soerjomataram, I.; Siegel, R.L.; Torre, L.A.; Jemal, A. Global cancer statistics 2018: GLOBOCAN estimates of incidence and mortality worldwide for 36 cancers in 185 countries. *CA A Cancer J. Clin.* **2018**, *68*, 394–424. [CrossRef] [PubMed]
2. Berger, M.D.; Ning, Y.; Stintzing, S.; Heinemann, V.; Cao, S.; Zhang, W.; Yang, D.; Miyamoto, Y.; Suenaga, M.; Schirripa, M.; et al. A polymorphism within the R-spondin 2 gene predicts outcome in metastatic colorectal cancer patients treated with FOLFIRI/bevacizumab: Data from FIRE-3 and TRIBE trials. *Eur. J. Cancer* **2020**, *131*, 89–97. [CrossRef] [PubMed]
3. Brenner, H.; Kloor, M.; Pox, C.P. Colorectal cancer. *Lancet* **2014**, *383*, 1490–1502. [CrossRef]
4. Gunderson, L.L.; Jessup, J.M.; Sargent, D.J.; Greene, F.L.; Stewart, A. Revised Tumor and Node Categorization for Rectal Cancer Based on Surveillance, Epidemiology, and End Results and Rectal Pooled Analysis Outcomes. *J. Clin. Oncol.* **2010**, *28*, 256–263. [CrossRef] [PubMed]
5. Tomlinson, J.S.; Jarnagin, W.R.; DeMatteo, R.P.; Fong, Y.; Kornprat, P.; Gonen, M.; Kemeny, N.; Brennan, M.F.; Blumgart, L.H.; D'Angelica, M. Actual 10-Year Survival After Resection of Colorectal Liver Metastases Defines Cure. *J. Clin. Oncol.* **2007**, *25*, 4575–4580. [CrossRef] [PubMed]
6. Argilés, G.; Tabernero, J.; Labianca, R.; Hochhauser, D.; Salazar, R.; Ivenson, T.; Laurent-Puig, P.; Quirke, P.; Yoshino, T.; Taieb, J.; et al. Localised colon cancer: ESMO Clinical Practice Guidelines for diagnosis, treatment and follow-up. *Ann. Oncol.* **2020**, *31*, 1291–1305. [CrossRef] [PubMed]
7. Shields, A.F. What is the optimal duration of adjuvant therapy in colon cancer? *Clin. Adv. Hematol. Oncol.* **2017**, *15*, 734–738.
8. Wyss, J.; Dislich, B.; Koelzer, V.H.; Galvan, J.A.; Dawson, H.; Hädrich, M.; Inderbitzin, D.; Lugli, A.; Zlobec, I.; Berger, M.D. Stromal PD-1/PD-L1 Expression Predicts Outcome in Colon Cancer Patients. *Clin. Color. Cancer* **2019**, *18*, e20–e38. [CrossRef]
9. Pagès, F.; Mlecnik, B.; Marliot, F.; Bindea, G.; Ou, F.S.; Bifulco, C.; Lugli, A.; Zlobec, I.; Rau, T.T.; Berger, M.D.; et al. International validation of the consensus Immunoscore for the classification of colon cancer: A prognostic and accuracy study. *Lancet* **2018**, *391*, 2128–2139. [CrossRef]
10. Li, Y.; Liang, L.; Dai, W.; Cai, G.; Xu, Y.; Li, X.; Li, Q.; Cai, S. Prognostic impact of programed cell death-1 (PD-1) and PD-ligand 1 (PD-L1) expression in cancer cells and tumor infiltrating lymphocytes in colorectal cancer. *Mol. Cancer* **2016**, *15*, 1–15. [CrossRef]
11. Andrews, L.P.; Marciscano, A.E.; Drake, C.G.; Vignali, D.A. LAG3 (CD223) as a cancer immunotherapy target. *Immunol. Rev.* **2017**, *276*, 80–96. [CrossRef] [PubMed]
12. Woo, S.R.; Turnis, M.E.; Goldberg, M.V.; Bankoti, J.; Selby, M.; Nirschl, C.J.; Bettini, M.L.; Gravano, D.M.; Vogel, P.; Liu, C.L.; et al. Immune inhibitory molecules LAG-3 and PD-1 synergistically regulate T-cell function to promote tumoral immune escape. *Cancer Res.* **2012**, *72*, 917–927. [CrossRef]
13. Kouo, T.; Huang, L.; Pucsek, A.B.; Cao, M.; Solt, S.; Amstrong, T.; Jaffee, E. Galectin-3 Shapes Antitumor Immune Responses by Suppressing CD8+ T Cells via LAG-3 and Inhibiting Expansion of Plasmacytoid Dendritic Cells. *Cancer Immunol. Res.* **2015**, *3*, 412–423. [CrossRef] [PubMed]
14. Long, L.; Zhang, X.; Chen, F.; Pan, Q.; Phiphatwatchara, P.; Zeng, Y.; Chen, H. The promising immune checkpoint LAG-3: From tumor microenvironment to cancer immunotherapy. *Genes Cancer* **2018**, *9*, 176–189. [CrossRef]
15. Xu, F.; Liu, J.; Liu, D.; Liu, B.; Wang, M.; Hu, Z.; Du, X.; Tang, L.; He, F. LSECtin Expressed on melanoma cells promotes tumor progression by inhibiting antitumor T-cell responses. *Cancer Res.* **2014**, *74*, 3418–3428. [CrossRef]
16. He, Y.; Rivard, C.J.; Rozeboom, L.; Yu, H.; Ellison, K.; Kowalewski, A.; Zhou, C.; Hirsch, F.R. Lymphocyte-activation gene-3, an important immune checkpoint in cancer. *Cancer Sci.* **2016**, *107*, 1193–1197. [CrossRef] [PubMed]
17. Ruffo, E.; Wu, R.C.; Bruno, T.C.; Workman, C.J.; Vignali, D.A.A. Lymphocyte-activation gene 3 (LAG3): The next immune checkpoint receptor. *Semin. Immunol.* **2019**, *42*, 101305. [CrossRef]
18. Dawson, H.; Galuppini, F.; Träger, P.; Berger, M.D.; Studer, P.; Brügger, L.; Zlobec, I.; Inderbitzin, D.; Lugli, A. Validation of the International Tumor Budding Consensus Conference 2016 recommendations on tumor budding in stage I-IV colorectal cancer. *Hum. Pathol.* **2019**, *85*, 145–151. [CrossRef]
19. Sobottka, B.; Moch, H.; Varga, Z. Differential PD-1/LAG-3 expression and immune phenotypes in metastatic sites of breast cancer. *Breast Cancer Res.* **2021**, *23*, 4. [CrossRef] [PubMed]
20. Interpretation Guide for Staining of Colorectal Tissue. Available online: https://diagnostics.roche.com/content/dam/diagnostics/us/en/products/c/colorectal-ihc-portfolio/MMR-IHC-Panel-InterpretationGuide.pdf (accessed on 3 July 2021).
21. Lee, S.J.; Jun, S.Y.; Lee, I.H.; Kang, B.W.; Park, S.Y.; Kim, H.J.; Park, J.S.; Choi, G.S.; Yoon, G.; Kim, J.G. CD274, LAG3, and IDO1 expressions in tumor-infiltrating immune cells as prognostic biomarker for patients with MSI-high colon cancer. *J. Cancer Res. Clin. Oncol.* **2018**, *144*, 1005–1014. [CrossRef] [PubMed]
22. Mlecnik, B.; Bindea, G.; Angell, H.K.; Maby, P.; Angelova, M.; Tougeron, D.; Church, S.E.; Lafontaine, L.; Fischer, M.; Fredriksen, T.; et al. Integrative analyses of colorectal cancer show Immunoscore is a stronger predictor of patient survival than microsatellite instability. *Immunity* **2016**, *44*, 698–711. [CrossRef]
23. Zhang, Y.; Liu, Y.; Luo, Y.; Liu, B.L.; Huang, Q.T.; Wang, F.; Zhong, Q. Prognostic value of Lymphocyte Activation Gene-3 (LAG-3) expression in esophageal squamous cell carcinoma. *J. Cancer* **2018**, *9*, 4287–4293. [CrossRef]
24. Hald, S.M.; Rakaee, M.; Martinez, I.; Richardsen, E.; Al-Saad, S.; Paulsen, E.E.; Blix, E.S.; Kilvaer, T.; Andersen, S.; Busund, L.T.; et al. LAG-3 in non–small-cell lung cancer: Expression in primary tumors and metastatic lymph nodes is associated with improved survival. *Clin. Lung Cancer* **2018**, *19*, 249–259.e2. [CrossRef]

25. Burugu, S.; Gao, D.; Leung, S.; Chia, S.K.; Nielsen, T.O. LAG-3+ tumor infiltrating lymphocytes in breast cancer: Clinical correlates and association with PD-1/PD-L1+ tumors. *Ann. Oncol.* **2017**, *28*, 2977–2984. [CrossRef] [PubMed]
26. Chen, J.; Chen, Z. The effect of immune microenvironment on the progression and prognosis of colorectal cancer. *Med. Oncol.* **2014**, *31*, 82. [CrossRef] [PubMed]
27. Saleh, R.; Taha, R.Z.; Toor, S.M.; Sasidharan Nair, V.; Murshed, K.; Khawar, M.; Al-Dhaheri, M.; Petkar, M.A.; Abu Nada, M.; Elkord, E. Expression of immune checkpoints and T cell exhaustion markers in early and advanced stages of colorectal cancer. *Cancer Immunol. Immunother.* **2020**, *69*, 1989–1999. [CrossRef]
28. Toor, S.M.; Murshed, K.; Al-Dhaheri, M.; Khawar, M.; Abu Nada, M.; Elkord, E. Immune Checkpoints in Circulating and Tumor-Infiltrating CD4+ T Cell Subsets in Colorectal Cancer Patients. *Front. Immunol.* **2019**, *10*, 2936. [CrossRef] [PubMed]
29. Larkin, J.; Chiarion-Sileni, V.; Gonzalez, R.; Grob, J.J.; Cowey, C.L.; Lao, C.D.; Schadendorf, D.; Dummer, R.; Smylie, M.; Rutkowski, P.; et al. Combined nivolumab and ipilimumab or monotherapy in untreated Melanoma. *N. Engl. J. Med.* **2015**, *373*, 23–34. [CrossRef]
30. Brahmer, J.; Reckamp, K.L.; Baas, P.; Crinò, L.; Eberhardt, W.E.; Poddubskaya, E.; Antonia, S.; Pluzanski, A.; Vokes, E.E.; Holgado, E.; et al. Nivolumab versus docetaxel in advanced squamous-cell non–small-cell lung cancer. *N. Engl. J. Med.* **2015**, *373*, 123–135. [CrossRef]
31. Motzer, R.J.; Escudier, B.; McDermott, D.F.; George, S.; Hammers, H.J.; Srinivas, S.; Tykodi, S.S.; Sosman, J.A.; Procopio, G.; Plimack, E.R.; et al. Nivolumab versus everolimus in advanced renal-cell carcinoma. *N. Engl. J. Med.* **2015**, *373*, 1803–1813. [CrossRef]
32. Bellmunt, J.; de Wit, R.; Vaughn, D.J.; Fradet, Y.; Lee, J.L.; Fong, L.; Vogelzang, N.J.; Climent, M.A.; Petrylak, D.P.; Choueiri, T.K.; et al. Pembrolizumab as second-line therapy for advanced urothelial carcinoma. *N. Engl. J. Med.* **2017**, *376*, 1015–1026. [CrossRef] [PubMed]
33. Ferris, R.L.; Blumenschein, G., Jr.; Fayette, J.; Guigay, J.; Colevas, A.D.; Licitra, L.; Harrington, K.; Kasper, S.; Vokes, E.E.; Even, C.; et al. Nivolumab for recurrent squamous-cell carcinoma of the head and neck. *N. Engl. J. Med.* **2016**, *375*, 1856–1867. [CrossRef] [PubMed]
34. Younes, A.; Santoro, A.; Shipp, M.; Zinzani, P.L.; Timmerman, J.M.; Ansell, S.; Armand, P.; Fanale, M.; Ratanatharathorn, V.; Kuruvilla, J.; et al. Nivolumab for classical Hodgkin's lymphoma after failure of both autologous stem-cell transplantation and brentuximab vedotin: A multicentre, multicohort, single-arm phase 2 trial. *Lancet Oncol.* **2016**, *17*, 1283–1294. [CrossRef]
35. Maruhashi, T.; Sugiura, D.; Okazaki, I.M.; Okazaki, T. LAG-3: From molecular functions to clinical applications. *J. Immunother. Cancer* **2020**, *8*, e001014. [CrossRef] [PubMed]
36. Lythgoe, M.P.; Liu, D.S.K.; Annels, N.E.; Krell, J.; Frampton, A.E. Gene of the month: Lymphocyte-activation gene 3 (LAG-3). *J. Clin. Pathol.* **2021**, *28*. [CrossRef]
37. Overman, M.J.; McDermott, R.; Leach, J.L.; Lonardi, S.; Lenz, H.J.; Morse, M.A.; Desai, J.; Hill, A.; Axelson, M.; Moss, R.A.; et al. Nivolumab in patients with metastatic DNA mismatch repair-deficient or microsatellite instability-high colorectal cancer (CheckMate 142): An open-label, multicentre, phase 2 study. *Lancet Oncol.* **2017**, 181182–181191. [CrossRef]
38. André, T.; Shiu, K.K.; Kim, T.W.; Jensen, B.V.; Jensen, L.H.; Punt, C.; Smith, D.; Garcia-Carbonero, R.; Benavides, M.; Gibbs, P.; et al. Pembrolizumab in microsatellite instability-high advanced colorectal cancer. *N. Engl. J. Med.* **2020**, *383*, 2207–2218. [CrossRef]
39. Eng, C.; Kim, T.W.; Bendell, J.; Argilés, G.; Tebbutt, N.C.; Di Bartolomeo, M.; Falcone, A.; Fakih, M.; Kozloff, M.; Segal, N.H.; et al. Atezolizumab with or without cobimetinib versus regorafenib in previously treated metastatic colorectal cancer (IMblaze370): A multicentre, open-label, phase 3, randomised, controlled trial. *Lancet Oncol.* **2019**, *20*, 849–861. [CrossRef]
40. Combination Chemotherapy with or without Atezolizumab in Treating Patients with Stage III Colon Cancer and Deficient DNA Mismatch Repair. Available online: https://clinicaltrials.gov/ct2/show/NCT02912559 (accessed on 25 January 2021).
41. Lau, D.; Kalaitzaki, E.; Church, D.N.; Pandha, H.; Tomlinson, I.; Annels, N.; Gerlinger, M.; Sclafani, F.; Smith, G.; Begum, R.; et al. Rationale and design of the POLEM trial: Avelumab plus fluoropyrimidine-based chemotherapy as adjuvant treatment for stage III mismatch repair deficient or POLE exonuclease domain mutant colon cancer: A phase III randomised study. *ESMO Open* **2020**, *5*, e000638. [CrossRef]

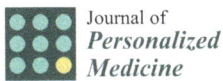

Article

Increased Expression of *VANGL1* Is Predictive of Lymph Node Metastasis in Colorectal Cancer: Results from a 20-Gene Expression Signature

Noshad Peyravian [1], Stefania Nobili [2], Zahra Pezeshkian [1], Meysam Olfatifar [1], Afshin Moradi [3], Kaveh Baghaei [1], Fakhrosadat Anaraki [4], Kimia Nazari [1], Hamid Asadzadeh Aghdaei [1], Mohammad Reza Zali [5], Enrico Mini [6,*] and Ehsan Nazemalhosseini Mojarad [5,*]

1. Basic and Molecular Epidemiology of Gastrointestinal Disorders Research Center, Research Institute for Gastroenterology and Liver Diseases, Shahid Beheshti University of Medical Sciences, Tehran 19875-17411, Iran; n.peyravian@gmail.com (N.P.); zahrapezeshkian@yahoo.com (Z.P.); ol.meysam92@gmail.com (M.O.); kavehbaghai@gmail.com (K.B.); k.nazari.1389@gmail.com (K.N.); hamid.assadzadeh@gmail.com (H.A.A.)
2. Department of Neurosciences, Imaging and Clinical Sciences, "G. D'Annunzio" University of Chieti-Pescara, 66100 Chieti, Italy; stefania.nobili@unich.it
3. Department of Pathology, Shohada Hospital, Shahid Beheshti University of Medical Sciences, Tehran 19875-17411, Iran; afshinmo2002@gmail.com
4. Colorectal Division of Department of Surgery, Taleghani Hospital, Shahid Beheshti University of Medical Sciences, Tehran 19875-17411, Iran; dr.anaraki47@gmail.com
5. Gastroenterology and Liver Diseases Research Center, Research Institute for Gastroenterology and Liver Diseases, Shahid Beheshti University of Medical Sciences, Yaman Street, Chamran Expressway, Tehran 19857-17411, Iran; nn.zali@hotmail.com
6. Department of Health Sciences, University of Florence, Viale Pieraccini 6, 50139 Firenze, Italy
* Correspondence: enrico.mini@unifi.it (E.M.); ehsanmojarad@gmail.com or E.nazemalhosseini@sbmu.ac.ir (E.N.M.)

Citation: Peyravian, N.; Nobili, S.; Pezeshkian, Z.; Olfatifar, M.; Moradi, A.; Baghaei, K.; Anaraki, F.; Nazari, K.; Aghdaei, H.A.; Zali, M.R.; et al. Increased Expression of *VANGL1* Is Predictive of Lymph Node Metastasis in Colorectal Cancer: Results from a 20-Gene Expression Signature. *J. Pers. Med.* **2021**, *11*, 126. https://doi.org/10.3390/jpm11020126

Academic Editor: Lisa Salvatore

Received: 26 December 2020
Accepted: 7 February 2021
Published: 14 February 2021

Publisher's Note: MDPI stays neutral with regard to jurisdictional claims in published maps and institutional affiliations.

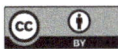

Copyright: © 2021 by the authors. Licensee MDPI, Basel, Switzerland. This article is an open access article distributed under the terms and conditions of the Creative Commons Attribution (CC BY) license (https://creativecommons.org/licenses/by/4.0/).

Abstract: This study aimed at building a prognostic signature based on a candidate gene panel whose expression may be associated with lymph node metastasis (LNM), thus potentially able to predict colorectal cancer (CRC) progression and patient survival. The mRNA expression levels of 20 candidate genes were evaluated by RT-qPCR in cancer and normal mucosa formalin-fixed paraffin-embedded (FFPE) tissues of CRC patients. Receiver operating characteristic curves were used to evaluate the prognosis performance of our model by calculating the area under the curve (AUC) values corresponding to stage and metastasis. A total of 100 FFPE primary tumor tissues from stage I–IV CRC patients were collected and analyzed. Among the 20 candidate genes we studied, only the expression levels of *VANGL1* significantly varied between patients with and without LNMs ($p = 0.02$). Additionally, the AUC value of the 20-gene panel was found to have the highest predictive performance (i.e., AUC = 79.84%) for LNMs compared with that of two subpanels including 5 and 10 genes. According to our results, *VANGL1* gene expression levels are able to estimate LNMs in different stages of CRC. After a proper validation in a wider case series, the evaluation of *VANGL1* gene expression and that of the 20-gene panel signature could help in the future in the prediction of CRC progression.

Keywords: colorectal cancer; gene signature; mRNA expression; *VANGL1*; FFPE

1. Introduction

Radical surgery and adjuvant chemotherapy improve the clinical outcome of stage III and high-risk stage II colorectal cancer (CRC) patients. However, it is known that 5-year overall survival (OS) highly varies according to important prognostic factors, such the pTs stage (stages II and III) and the involvement of lymph nodes (pN1 and pN2 stage III) [1–3]. Overall, lymph node metastasis (LNM) is a key prognostic factor for the determination of

CRC outcomes and significantly relates to poorer prognosis, disease-free survival (DFS), and OS [4,5].

Available clinical data suggest that the accurate diagnosis of LNM is not only important for the prediction of the prognosis of patients but also useful for further therapeutic management, such as for the selection of patients who would benefit from adjuvant/neoadjuvant chemotherapy or chemo-radiotherapy [2,6,7]. In fact, the number and sites of lymph nodes involved have a direct impact on the stage of disease as established by the AJCC tumor-node-metastasis (TNM) staging classification for colon cancer [8].

However, it should be noted that pathological methods are not able to diagnose occult LNMs (micrometastases). Thus, the use of advanced methodologies (e.g., gene expression profiling (GEP)), the investigation of specific biomarkers (e.g., microsatellite instability (MSI)), CpG island methylator phenotype (CIMP), the application of the immune score recommended for increasing the detection power of disease recurrence, and in this regard the use of genes associated with lymph node involvement are very useful to enhance this evaluation [9–12]. In this regard, GEP has been used to discover biomarkers associated with lymph nodes in epithelial neoplasms, such as pancreatic cancer [13], oral squamous cell carcinoma [14], invasive breast cancer [15], and CRC [16]. However, the power of diagnosis may vary based on gene selection.

High-throughput studies in which biomarkers of tumor suppressor genes and oncogenes are potentially able to predict the prognosis of CRC patients at different stages of disease and according to the lymph node involvement are available [4,8,17].

In order to find a suitable biomarker to predict LNM involvement, we evaluated gene expression profiling studies and selected 20 genes (*VANGL1, SMAD2, BUB1, EGFR, HES1, MAP2K1, NOTCH1, ANXA3, SMAD4, MTA1, LEF1, RHOA, TGF-ß, CD44, CD133, IL2RA, IL2RB, PITX2, PCSK7*, and *FOLH1*) that play a key role in carcinogenesis, tumor growth, LNM development tumor invasion, and metastasis by regulating a variety of cellular processes (Table 1) [4,16–20].

Table 1. Information * on the biological functions of 20 candidate genes and on the primer sequences used for RT-qPCR

Gene Symbol	Gene Name and Functions	Primer Sequence
VANGL1 (KITENIN)	VANGL planar cell polarity protein 1 (located on chromosome 1) 1. It encodes a member of the tetraspanin family. 2. It may be involved in mediating intestinal trefoil factor-induced wound healing in the intestinal mucosa.	F: 5′-GACACAAGTCACCCCGGAATA-3′ R: 5′-TCCTCTGTCCGAGTAGAATCATT-3′ Amplicon length: 109 bp
IL2RA (CD25)	Interleukin 2 receptor subunit alpha (located on chromosome 10) 1. Mutations in this gene are associated with interleukin 2 receptor alpha deficiency. 2. Serum IL-2R levels are found to be elevated in patients with different types of carcinomas.	F: 5′-GAACACAACGAAACAAGTGACAC-3′ R: 5′-GGCTGCATTGGACTTTGCATT-3′ Amplicon length: 81 bp
IL2RB (CD122)	Interleukin 2 receptor subunit beta (located on chromosome 22) 1. It is involved in receptor-mediated endocytosis and transduction of mitogenic signals from IL2.	F: 5′-CAGCGGTGAATGGCACTTC-3′ R: 5′-GGCATGGACTTGGCAGGAA-3′ Amplicon length: 113 bp
TGFβ1	Transforming growth factor ß (located on chromosome 19) 1. It encodes a secreted ligand of the TGFß superfamily of proteins. The encoded protein regulates cell proliferation, differentiation, and growth. 2. It is frequently upregulated in tumor cells.	F: 5′-CAATTCCTGGCGATACCTCAG-3′ R: 5′-GCACAACTCCGGTGACATCAA-3′ Amplicon length: 86 bp
SMAD2	SMAD2 family member 2 (located on chromosome 18) 1. The protein encoded mediates the signal of the transforming growth factor (TGF)-beta, thus regulating multiple cellular processes (i.e., cell proliferation, apoptosis, and differentiation).	F: 5′-CCGACACACCGAGATCCTAAC-3′ R: 5′-GAGGTGGCGTTTCTGGAATATAA-3′ Amplicon length: 125 bp
SMAD4	SMAD4 family member 4 (Located on chromosome 18) 1. The encoded protein forms homomeric complexes and heteromeric complexes with other activated Smad proteins that accumulate in the nucleus and regulate the transcription of target genes. 2. The encoded protein acts as a tumor suppressor and inhibits epithelial cell proliferation.	F: 5′-CCACCAAGTAATCGTGCATCG-3′ R: 5′-TGGTAGCATTAGACTCAGATGGG-3′ Amplicon length: 76 bp

Table 1. Cont.

Gene Symbol	Gene Name and Functions	Primer Sequence
CD44 (CSPG8)	CD44 antigen (located on chromosome 11) 1. It is a cell-surface glycoprotein involved in cell–cell interactions, cell adhesion, and migration. 2. The encoded protein participates in several cellular functions (e.g., lymphocyte activation, recirculation and homing, hematopoiesis, and tumor metastasis).	F: 5′-CTGCCGCTTTGCAGGTGTA-3′ R: 5′-CATTGTGGGCAAGGTGCTATT-3′ Amplicon length: 109 bp
CD133 (PROM1)	CD133 (located on chromosome 4) 1. It encodes a pentaspan transmembrane glycoprotein. 2. The encoded protein is often expressed on adult stem cells, where it has been suggested to maintain stem cell properties by suppressing differentiation. 3. It is the marker most commonly used for the isolation of cancer stem cell population from different tumors.	F: 5′-GGCCCAGTACAACACTACCAA-3′ R: 5′-ATTCCGCCTCCTAGCACTGAA-3′ Amplicon length: 75 bp
HES1	HES family basic helix-loop-helix (bHLH) transcription factor 1 (chromosome 3) 1. It is a transcriptional repressor of genes that require a bHLH protein for their transcription. 2. It plays an important role in the Notch signaling pathway. 3. The absence of Hes1 in the developing intestine promotes the increase of Math1 (the production of intestinal cell types).	F: 5′-ACGTGCGAGGGCGTTAATAC-3′ R: 5′-GGGGTAGGTCATGGCATTGA-3′ Amplicon length: 90 bp
NOTCH1	NOTCH receptor 1 (located on chromosome 9) 1. The Notch signaling pathway regulates interactions between physically adjacent cells through the binding of Notch family receptors to their cognate ligands. 2. It plays a role in the development of numerous cell and tissue types. 3. Mutations in NOTCH1 are associated with syndromes, hematological and solid tumors.	F: 5′-TGGACCAGATTGGGGAGTTC-3′ R: 5′-GCACACTCGTCTGTGTTGAC-3′ Amplicon length: 82 bp
LEF1 (TCF10)	Lymphoid enhancer-binding factor 1 (located on chromosome 4) 1. It encodes a transcription factor belonging to a family of proteins that share homology with the high mobility group protein-1. 2. It binds to a functionally important site in the T-cell receptor-alpha (TCRA) enhancer, thus conferring maximal enhancer activity. 3. It is involved in the Wnt signaling pathway, and mutations in this gene have been found in some tumors.	F: 5′-ATGTCAACTCCAAACAAGGCA-3′ R: 5′-CCCGGAGACAAGGGATAAAAAGT-3′ Amplicon length: 76 bp
MTA1	Metastasis-associated 1 (located on chromosome 14) 1. MTA1 expression has been correlated with the metastatic potential of some carcinomas, but it is expressed also in many normal tissues. 2. The profile and activity of the encoded protein suggest that it is involved in regulating transcription and that this may be accomplished by chromatin remodeling.	F: 5′-ACGCAACCCTGTCAGTCTG-3′ R: 5′-GGGCAGGTCCACCATTTCC-3′ Amplicon length: 104 bp
EGFR (ErBb-1)	Epidermal growth factor receptor (located on chromosome 7) 1. It encodes a transmembrane glycoprotein that is a member of the protein kinase (PK) superfamily. 2. EGFR binds to EGF, thus inducing receptor dimerization and tyrosine autophosphorylation, leading to cell proliferation. 3. Mutations in EGFR are associated with lung cancer.	F: 5′-TGCGTCTCTTGCCGGAAT-3′ R: 5′-GGCTCACCCTCCAGAAGGTT-3′ Amplicon length: 71 bp
MAP2K1 (MEK1)	Mitogen-activated protein kinase kinase 1 (located on chromosome 15) 1. The encoded protein is a member of the dual specificity PK family that acts as a mitogen-activated protein (MAP) kinase kinase. 2. The encoded protein stimulates the enzymatic activity of MAP kinases upon a wide variety of extra- and intracellular signals. 3. As a component of the MAP kinase signal transduction pathway, the encoded protein is involved in many cellular processes (e.g., proliferation, differentiation, and transcription regulation).	F: 5′-CAATGGCGGTGTGGTGTTC-3′ R: 5′-GATTGCGGGTTTGATCTCCAG-3′ Amplicon length: 91 bp
FOLH1 (PSMA)	Folate hydrolase 1 (located on chromosome 11) 1. It encodes a type II transmembrane glycoprotein belonging to the M28 peptidase family. 2. Also known as prostate-specific membrane antigen (PSMA), it is expressed in many tissues, including the prostate. 3. In the prostate, the FOLH1/PSMA protein is upregulated in cancer cells and is used as an effective diagnostic and prognostic indicator of prostate cancer.	F: 5′-AGAGGGCGATCTAGTGTATGTT-3′ R: 5′-TGATTTTCATGTCCCGTTCCAAT-3′ Amplicon length: 74 bp

Table 1. Cont.

Gene Symbol	Gene Name and Functions	Primer Sequence
BUB1	BUB1 mitotic checkpoint serine/threonine kinase (located on chromosome 2) 1. It encodes a protein that plays a central role in mitosis. 2. This protein may also function in the DNA damage response. 3. Mutations in this gene have been associated with aneuploidy and several forms of cancer.	F: 5′-AGCCCAGACAGTAACAGACTC-3′ R: 5′-GTTGGCAACCTTATGTGTTTCAC-3′ Amplicon length: 136 bp
RHOA	Ras homolog family member A (located on chromosome 3) 1. It encodes a member of the Rho family of small GTPases that function as molecular switches in signal transduction cascades. 2. Overexpression of this gene is associated with tumor cell proliferation and metastasis.	F: 5′-GGAAAGCAGGTAGAGTTGGCT-3′ R: 5′-GGCTGTCGATGGAAAAACACAT-3′ Amplicon length: 118 bp
PCSK7	Proprotein convertase subtilisin/kexin type 7 (located on chromosome 11) 1. It encodes a type 1 membrane-bound protease that is expressed in many tissues, including the neuroendocrine, liver, gut, and brain. 2. It has been implicated in the transcriptional regulation of housekeeping genes. 3. A chromosomal translocation associated with B-cell lymphoma occurs between this gene and its inverted counterpart.	F: 5′-GCAGCGTCCACTTCAACGA-3′ R: 5′-GCCCAGTCACATTGCGTTC-3′ Amplicon length: 117 bp
PITX2 (ARP1)	Paired-like homeodomain 2 (located on chromosome 4) 1. It encodes a member of the RIEG/PITX homeobox family, which is in the bicoid class of homeodomain proteins. 3. The encoded protein acts as a transcription factor and regulates procollagen lysyl hydroxylase gene expression.	F: 5′-GCCAAGGGCCTTACATCCG-3′ R: 5′-GGTGGGGAAAACATGCTCTG-3′ Amplicon length: 101 bp
ANXA3 (annexin) A3	Annexin A3 (located on chromosome 4) 1. It encodes a member of the annexin family. 1. Members of this calcium-dependent phospholipid-binding protein family play a role in the regulation of cellular growth and in signal transduction pathways. 2. The encoded protein functions in the inhibition of phospholipase A2 and cleavage of inositol 1,2-cyclic phosphate to form inositol 1-phosphate.	F: 5′-TTAGCCCATCAGTGGATGCTG-3′ R: 5′-CTGTGCATTTGACCTCTCAGT-3′ Amplicon length: 104 bp
B2M	β2-microglobulin (located on chromosome 15) – Housekeeping gene	F: 5′-TGCTGTCTCCATGTTTGATGTATCT-3′ R: 5′-TCTCTGCTCCCCACCTCTAAGT-3′ Amplicon length: 86 bp
ACTB	β-actin (located on chromosome 7) – Housekeeping gene	F: 5′- GCCGGGACCTGACTGACTAC-3′ R: 5′- TTCTCCTTAATGTCACGCACGAT-3′ Amplicon length: 100 bp

* Information available at https://www.ncbi.nlm.nih.gov/ (accessed on 10 February 2021).

Thus, the aim of this study was to identify at the mRNA level and to validate at the protein level the potential prognostic role of these candidate genes in relation to the LNM of CRC patients.

2. Materials and Methods

2.1. Patients and Sample Collection

This retrospective study was performed in 100 formalin-fixed paraffin-embedded (FFPE) tumor tissues of CRC patients at stage I or II ($n = 52$) and at stage III or IV ($n = 48$) and 10 FFPE samples of normal tissues (colonic mucosa) as calibrators in RT-qPCR, as well as paired samples of normal colonic tissues from the same CRC patients. All samples were anonymized. Patients underwent surgical resection for CRC from February 1998 to December 2018 at Taleghani Hospital, Shahid Beheshti University of Medical Sciences, Tehran, Iran. They were chemo- and radiotherapy naïve, and none of them experienced previous neoplastic disease. Clinical information, such as colonoscopy/pathology report, follow-up data, and cause of death, was collected from medical records. All patients were carefully followed up to confirm their clinical outcomes.

This study was approved by the ethical committee (IR.SBMU.RIGLD.REC.1396.947) of the Research Institute for Gastroenterology and Liver Disease, Shahid Beheshti University of Medical Sciences, Tehran, Iran. Written informed consent was obtained from all patients.

The inclusion criteria for the patients were the following: (1) signed informed consent; (2) availability of the pathology report to confirm the tumor histology; (3) nonresident in an institution, such as a prison, nursing home, or shelter; (4) no severe illness in the intensive care unit; and (5) no preoperative chemotherapy and radiotherapy. The exclusion criteria were the following: patients affected by familial adenomatous polyposis (FAP), hereditary nonpolyposis CRC (HNPCC), cancer at any site at the time of selection, and patients who received neoadjuvant chemotherapy or radiotherapy. The FFPE tissue blocks were cut 10–15 μm and 4–7 μm in thickness for mRNA extraction and immunohistochemistry (IHC), respectively.

To ensure the quality of the presence of tumor and normal cells in FFPE tissue blocks, before performing the laboratory process, each section was evaluated for tumor and normal cells (>80% representative) by the pathologist using hematoxylin and eosin (H&E) staining.

2.2. RNA Isolation

Ten–fifteen micrometer thick sections were cut from the FFPE blocks, and each section was transferred into a microcentrifuge tube. Deparaffinization was performed with 1 mL xylene, incubating twice for 10 min, and 1 mL absolute ethanol, also incubating twice for 10 min.

2.3. Quantitative and Qualitative Analysis of the Isolated RNA Samples

Total RNA was extracted from the target tissues using the Rneasy Kit (Qiagen, Chatsworth, CA) according to the company's protocol. To avoid genomic DNA contamination, RNA samples were treated with Dnase I according to the manufacturer's protocol (Invitrogen, Carlsbad, CA, USA). RNA concentration was measured by a NanoDrop ND-1000 spectrophotometer (NanoDrop Technologies Inc., Rockland, DE, USA). An A260/A280 ratio was used to evaluate the RNA purity, and values in the range of 1.8–2.0 were accepted.

2.4. Real-Time PCR Analysis

cDNAs were generated with a PrimeScript RT Reagent kit (Takara, Shiga, Japan) according to the manufacturer's protocol.

The mRNA levels of 20 candidate genes (i.e., *VANGL1, IL2RA, IL2RB, TGF-β, SMAD2, SMAD4, CD44, CD133, HES1, NOTCH1, LEF1, MTA1, EGFR, MAP2K1, FOLH1, BUB1, RHOA1, PCSK7, PITX2*, and *ANXA3*) (Table 1) and of the housekeeping gene β2-microglobulin (*B2M*) were analyzed by RT-qPCR using the SYBR Fast qPCR Mix Kit (Takara). The cDNA samples were amplified by the 7500 Real-Time PCR System (Applied Biosystems, Foster City, CA, USA) with an initial denaturation at 95 °C for 30 s, followed by 40 cycles each at 95 °C for 5 s and 60 °C for 34 s. Relative expression abundances of the target genes were determined by normalizing to *B2M* and *β-actin* using the $2^{-\Delta\Delta Ct}$ method. Each measurement was performed in triplicate. *B2M* was utilized to calculate the relative quantitation (RQ) of mRNA transcripts using the $2^{-\Delta\Delta Ct}$ method.

2.5. Unsupervised Hierarchical Clustering

An unsupervised hierarchical clustering was used to graphically display the expression levels of 20 candidate genes in CRC samples. Dendrograms and clustering were generated by using the Gene Cluster version 3.0 software and visualized with the Java TreeView version 3.0, available at http://rana.lbl.gov/EisenSoftware.htm (accessed on 1 February 2021) and http://jtreeview.sourceforge.net (accessed on 1 February 2021), respectively. The color of each square box represents the ratio of gene expression. Green boxes indicate upregulated genes, while red boxes represent downregulated genes.

2.6. Immunohistochemistry and Evaluation of Staining

To investigate the expression levels of candidate proteins, an IHC analysis was performed on slices of FFPE tissues ranging from 4 to 7 μm in thickness. For deparaffinization, the slides were incubated at 37 °C for 24 h and then washed with xylene (100%), ethanol (100%, 85%, and 75%), and distilled water, respectively. After deparaffinization, slides were incubated in a solution of 10% H_2O_2 and methanol at a ratio of 1:9 for 15 min and subsequently washed with the distilled water. Next, the slides were treated in the 10 mM citrate buffer solution (pH = 6) and microwaved with 800 W for 24 min and washed with the Tris-buffered saline (TBS). After treating with the blocking serum for 15 min, the slides were immunostained with mouse anti-human MoAbs for 45 min and later washed with TBS. Later, by treating with the EnVision + visualization system (Dako) for 30 min, followed by DAB (Master Diagnosis, LOT. No 090517C1-01) as the chromogen substrate for 10 min, the bound primary antibody was visualized. Finally, the slides were washed with distilled water, dehydrated with ethanol, and stained in hematoxylin. All the slides were independently checked by investigators who had no knowledge of the patients' characteristics and clinical outcome using a microscope (Nikon, Tokyo, Japan).

The analysis of immunostaining intensity was performed using a qualitative scale and ocular observation. Sections were first scanned at low-power magnification (10x) and were quantitatively assessed as follows: under a light microscope at 400x magnifications, five high-power fields (HPFs) were randomly selected, and the immunostaining intensity was determined.

Mean values were estimated through the scanning of the entire tissue sections of all samples using two graded scales: negative, <10%, and positive, >10%. The positive controls were the following: (a) a normal colonic tissue was taken as an internal control for ß-catenin IHC, and (b) a histologically diagnosed section of colon carcinoma tissues for nuclear positivity by ß-catenin IHC. Negative control was achieved by omitting the primary antibody. The MoAbs used in this study were VANGL1 (Abcam, Anti-VANGL1 antibody ab69227), SMAD4 (Abcam, Phospho-SMAD4 antibody T277), EGFR (Master Diagnosis, Anti-EGFR antibody Lot No. 0664000), and LEF1 (Master Diagnosis, Anti-EGFR antibody Lot No. 07430003).

2.7. Statistical Analysis

Tumors were divided into lymph node metastases (LNMs) and non-lymph node metastases (non-LNMs) based on the histopathological results. The mRNA expression levels of tumor tissues were represented as the mean ± standard deviation (SD). The Mann–Whitney U and Kruskal–Wallis tests were used to assess the differences of the mRNA expressions of 20 genes between the established groups (i.e., presence/absence of LNMs; stage (I–II vs. III–IV), tumor differentiation grade (well vs. poor differentiated), sex (male vs. female), and age (<50 vs. ≥50)). All statistical analyses were performed by the IBM SPSS Statistics software version 22 (IBM, SPSS, Chicago, IL, USA) and Stata analyzer.

For receiver operating characteristic (ROC) curve analysis, the R 3.6.1 software was used to evaluate the sensitivity and specificity of the prognosis prediction (evaluated by OS) according to the mRNA gene expression by analyzing the area under the curve (AUC). Stratification of patients in high and low tumor gene expression was established according to the cutoff obtained for each gene by ROC analysis. OS analysis was performed by plotting Kaplan–Meier (log-rank test) curves. p-Values < 0.05 were considered statistically significant.

3. Results

3.1. Clinical and Pathological Characteristics of Patients

The population study consisted of 100 FFPE tissues from CRC patients (59 men and 41 women with an average age of 52.17 years, 20–78 range). The clinical features of the study population are shown in Table 2. Information on age, sex, stage, tumor differentiation, and tumor location is available for all patients. Among patients, 52% had stage I or II CRC, while 48% of the cases had stage III or IV. Of 100 patients, 37 were positive and 63 were negative for LNM.

Table 2. Clinical and pathological characteristics of patients.

Characteristics	Number of Patients, 100 (%)
Gender	
Male	59 (59%)
Female	41 (41%)
Age	
<50 years	59 (59%)
≥50 years	41 (41%)
Tumor localization	
Left (descending colon)	49 (49%)
Right (ascending colon)	51 (51%)
Tumor stage	
I	9 (9%)
II	43 (43%)
III	41 (41%)
IV	7 (7%)
Differentiation grade	
Well differentiated	82 (82%)
Poorly differentiated	18 (18%)
Lymph node metastasis	
Yes	37 (37%)
No	63 (63%)
Median overall survival, range	10.8 years, 0.019–21 years

3.2. Gene Expression Analysis

To identify molecular determinants of LNMs, gene expression profiles from patients with or without LNMs and at different stages of disease were compared. Based on literature data, we selected 20 genes that relate to the lymphatic metastatic process and evaluated their expression levels in 100 FFPE blocks.

Relationships of tumor gene expression with demographic (sex, age), clinical (tumor location), and pathological (stage, LNM, grade) features are reported in Tables 3 and 4.

Table 3. Relationships between the expression of 20 CRC study genes and age and sex.

Gene Symbol	Fold Change of Age			Fold Change of Sex		
	<50	≥50	p-Value	Male	Female	p-Value
VANGL1	4.910 ± 7.56	7.155 ± 10.54	0.44	5.706 ± 9.02	6.972 ± 10.08	0.36
IL2RA	0.603 ± 0.640	1.509 ± 1.83	0.02	1.148 ± 1.61	1.098 ± 1.37	0.93
IL2RB	0.699 ± 1.10	0.635 ± 1.24	0.88	0.870 ± 1.37	0.351 ± 0.71	0.02
TGFβ	1.056 ± 1.61	1.285 ± 2.02	0.79	1.308 ± 2.14	1.010 ± 1.34	0.90
SMAD2	1.313 ± 2.20	0.855 ± 1.45	0.74	0.942 ± 1.64	1.205 ± 2.06	0.30
SMAD4	2.157 ± 2.36	2.425 ± 2.21	0.41	2.417 ± 2.20	2.157 ± 2.37	0.34
CD44	0.596 ± 0.814	0.537 ± 0.87	0.44	0.478 ± 0.85	0.687 ± 0.82	0.10
CD133	0.832 ± 1.77	1.329 ± 2.83	0.62	0.870 ± 2.43	1.495 ± 2.44	0.07
HES1	2.830 ± 3.52	2.134 ± 3.28	0.36	2.685 ± 3.39	0.955 ± 3.38	0.44
NOTCH1	1.088 ± 2.18	0.953 ± 2.22	0.58	0.795 ± 2.36	1.332 ± 1.89	0.02
LEF1	1.178 ± 1.80	1.038 ± 1.19	0.58	0.988 ± 1.14	1.260 ± 1.86	0.86
MTA1	1.045 ± 1.01	1.012 ± 0.98	0.85	0.947 ± 0.93	1.144 ± 1.06	0.37

Table 3. Cont.

Gene Symbol	Fold Change of Age			Fold Change of Sex		
	<50	≥50	p-Value	Male	Female	p-Value
EGFR	2.272 ± 2.60	2.937 ± 4.65	0.75	2.439 ± 3.43	2.986 ± 4.58	0.87
MAP2K1	1.722 ± 2.47	1.235 ± 2.23	0.02	1.495 ± 2.65	1.355 ± 1.78	0.49
FOLH1	0.797 ± 0.70	0.814 ± 0.91	0.65	0.809 ± 0.85	0.804 ± 0.81	0.78
BUB1	0.656 ± 1.65	0.610 ± 1.46	0.18	0.731 ± 1.53	0.476 ± 1.56	0.27
RHOA	0.510 ± 0.621	0.562 ± 1.19	0.11	0.625 ± 1.11	0.414 ± 0.75	0.50
PCSK7	6.590 ± 7.74	3.069 ± 4.48	0.19	4.196 ± 5.12	5.076 ± 6.02	0.42
PITX2	0.976 ± 2.00	0.663 ± 1.13	0.57	0.720 ± 1.13	0.906 ± 2.05	0.58
ANXA3	3.533 ± 4.70	4.399 ± 6.65	0.60	4.298 ± 6.06	3.641 ± 5.71	0.12

Table 4. Relationships between the expression of 20 CRC study genes and clinical and pathological characteristics of patients.

Gene Symbol	Fold Change of Stage			Fold Change of Lymph Node Metastasis			Fold Change of Tumor Site			Fold Change of Differentiation Grade		
	I, II	III, IV	p-Value	Yes	No	p-Value	Right	Left	p-Value	Well	Poor	p-Value
VANGL1	3.795 ± 5.63	8.831 ± 11.80	0.05	9.749 ± 12.40	4.136 ± 6.38	0.02	7.144 ± 10.44	5.243 ± 8.23	0.26	6.516 ± 9.22	4.831 ± 10.50	0.07
IL2RA	1.073 ± 1.59	1.188 ± 1.44	0.40	0.982 ± 1.19	1.214 ± 1.68	0.85	1.293 ± 1.84	0.957 ± 1.08	0.63	1.221 ± 1.56	0.707 ± 1.23	0.12
IL2RB	0.728 ± 1.31	0.591 ± 1.02	0.64	0.433 ± 0.43	0.797 ± 1.33	0.19	0.520 ± 0.85	0.811 ± 1.44	0.78	0.618 ± 1.21	0.864 ± 1.00	0.05
TGFβ	0.977 ± 1.50	1.418 ± 2.17	0.71	1.560 ± 2.25	0.971 ± 1.56	0.22	1.086 ± 1.66	1.296 ± 2.06	0.53	1.649 ± 1.84	1.088 ± 1.90	0.26
SMAD2	1.257 ± 2.13	0.821 ± 1.37	0.27	0.702 ± 1.26	1.250 ± 2.05	0.19	1.053 ± 2.17	1.043 ± 1.36	0.24	0.371 ± 1.95	1.196 ± 0.65	0.04
SMAD4	2.483 ± 2.50	2.128 ± 1.99	0.78	2.096 ± 1.99	2.440 ± 2.41	0.82	2.165 ± 2.41	2.467 ± 2.11	0.37	2.068 ± 2.20	2.367 ± 2.60	0.22
CD44	0.480 ± 0.61	0.650 ± 1.03	0.77	0.767 ± 1.14	0.441 ± 0.58	0.65	0.705 ± 1.03	0.413 ± 0.55	0.24	0.570 ± 0.76	0.522 ± 1.15	0.35
CD133	0.842 ± 1.99	1.421 ± 2.85	0.63	1.324 ± 2.43	1.000 ± 2.46	0.50	0.831 ± 1.59	1.421 ± 3.08	0.45	1.204 ± 2.63	0.738 ± 1.21	0.26
HES1	2.111 ± 2.96	2.767 ± 3.80	0.44	2.944 ± 4.06	2.123 ± 2.91	0.33	2.707 ± 3.90	2.134 ± 2.76	0.29	2.637 ± 3.58	1.465 ± 2.11	0.47
NOTCH1	1.147 ± 2.44	0.861 ± 1.90	0.66	0.968 ± 2.10	1.034 ± 2.26	0.87	0.768 ± 1.49	1.261 ± 2.73	0.16	1.170 ± 2.38	0.278 ± 0.49	0.13
LEF1	0.844 ± 0.87	1.371 ± 1.89	0.76	1.424 ± 1.99	0.905 ± 1.02	0.67	0.980 ± 1.49	1.218 ± 1.45	0.21	1.056 ± 1.34	1.283 ± 2.00	0.51
MTA1	0.983 ± 0.98	1.072 ± 1.00	0.72	1.073 ± 1.03	0.998 ± 0.96	0.83	1.178 ± 0.97	0.868 ± 0.99	0.08	1.024 ± 0.98	1.032 ± 1.04	0.89
EGFR	2.693 ± 3.86	2.620 ± 4.02	0.84	2.091 ± 2.65	2.990 ± 4.49	0.56	3.214 ± 4.31	2.078 ± 3.40	0.22	2.595 ± 4.12	2.945 ± 2.91	0.33
MAP2K1	1.442 ± 2.57	1.436 ± 2.07	0.33	1.549 ± 1.25	1.253 ± 2.58	0.98	1.251 ± 2.09	1.636 ± 2.57	0.34	1.377 ± 2.34	1.724 ± 2.34	0.39
FOLH1	0.857 ± 0.90	0.753 ± 0.75	0.55	0.767 ± 0.76	0.831 ± 0.87	0.79	0.848 ± 0.90	0.764 ± 0.75	0.70	0.829 ± 0.86	0.708 ± 0.67	0.83
BUB1	0.607 ± 1.35	0.652 ± 1.73	0.95	0.617 ± 1.67	0.636 ± 1.47	0.96	0.559 ± 1.28	0.702 ± 1.78	0.65	0.695 ± 1.68	0.328 ± 0.48	0.27
RHOA	0.294 ± 0.39	0.807 ± 1.32	0.21	0.916 ± 1.46	0.320 ± 0.43	0.24	0.645 ± 1.13	0.431 ± 0.81	0.36	0.501 ± 0.86	0.720 ± 1.44	0.78
PCSK7	4.290 ± 5.74	4.827 ± 6.81	0.12	4.170 ± 5.51	4.770 ± 6.21	0.19	3.614 ± 4.51	5.520 ± 6.32	0.07	4.364 ± 5.65	5.384 ± 6.96	1.00
PITX2	0.644 ± 1.03	0.957 ± 1.95	0.98	1.079 ± 2.16	0.627 ± 1.03	0.63	0.959 ± 1.98	0.622 ± 0.92	0.84	0.737 ± 1.12	1.056 ± 2.82	0.21
ANXA3	3.320 ± 4.54	4.811 ± 7.06	0.67	5.542 ± 7.75	3.150 ± 4.31	0.21	4.597 ± 7.06	3.450 ± 4.39	0.73	7.065 ± 4.91	3.370 ± 8.71	0.01

In particular, the gene expression levels of VANGL1 varied significantly between patients with and without LNMs. The tumors of patients with LNMs displayed twofold higher levels of *VANGL1* mRNA expression compared with those of patients without LNMs ($p = 0.02$) (Table 4 and Figure 1). Additionally, the expression levels of this gene varied between patients with stages I-II and III-IV, showing the highest mean level (i.e., 8.831) for stages III and IV. This difference reached a good level of significance, although not fully significant ($p = 0.05$) (Table 4 and Figure 1).

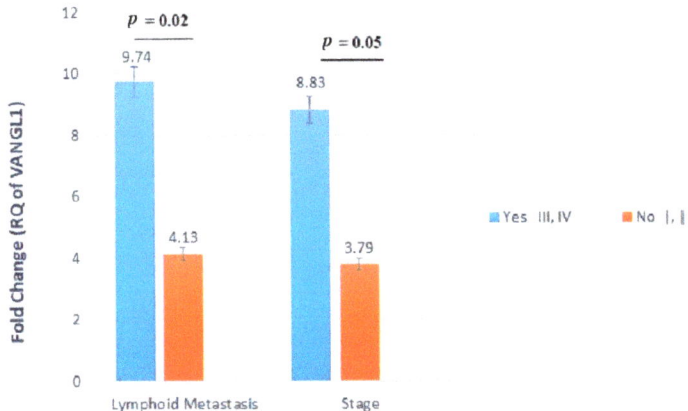

Figure 1. *VANGL1* mRNA relative quantification (RQ) established by RT-qPCR analysis according to lymph node metastasis (LNMs) involvement or stage. Gene expression levels of *VANGL1* differed significantly between patients with and without LNMs.

The mRNA expression levels of three genes (i.e., *IL2RB*, *SMAD*, and *ANXA3*) were significantly ($p < 0.05$) different between well-differentiated (i.e., G1 and G2) and poorly differentiated (i.e., G3 and G4) tumors (Table 4 and Figure 2).

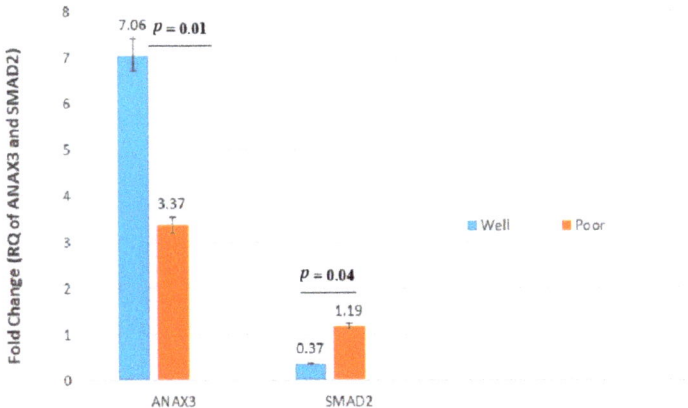

Figure 2. *ANXA3* and *SMAD2* mRNA relative quantification (RQ) established by RT-qPCR analysis according to histological grade. Gene expression levels of these genes differed significantly between well- and poorly differentiated cancers.

We found significant associations between tumor mRNA expression of *IL2RB* and *NOTCH1* genes and gender and between tumor mRNA expression of *IL2RA* and *MAP2K1* genes and age. In particular, the *IL2RA* gene was significantly downregulated in patients younger than 50 years old compared with patients older than 50 years (Figure 3). Additionally, an increased expression of the *MAP2K1* gene was observed in patients older than

50 years in comparison with patients younger than 50 years old ($p = 0.02$). *IL2RB* exhibited lower expression in females compared with males ($p = 0.02$) (Table 3 and Figure 4). Conversely, the *NOTCH1* gene was significantly upregulated in female patients as compared with male CRC cases ($p = 0.02$).

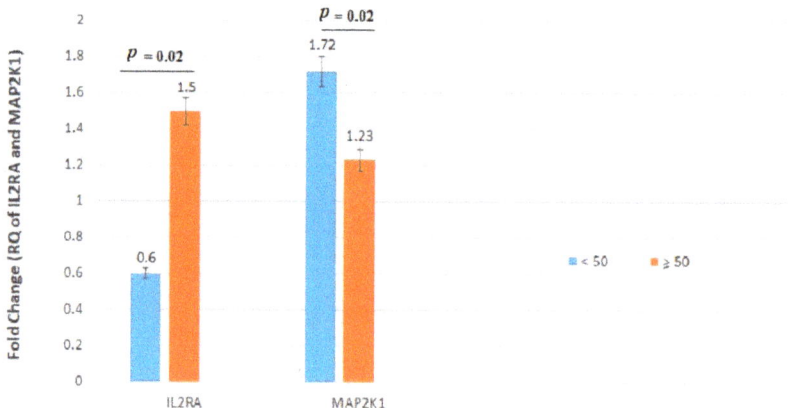

Figure 3. *IL2RA* and *MAP2K1* mRNA relative quantification established by RT-qPCR analysis according to age. Gene expression levels of these genes differed significantly between patients younger than 50 years and patients older than or equal to 50 years.

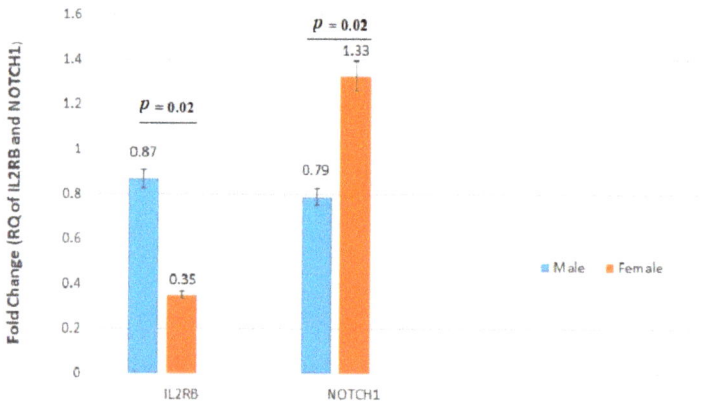

Figure 4. *IL2RB* and *NOTCH1* mRNA relative quantification (RQ) established by RT-qPCR analysis according to gender. Gene expression levels of these genes differed significantly between males and females.

3.3. Heat Maps of Real-Time PCR Data

Hierarchical clustering of 100 CRC samples is reported in Figure 5. According to the diagram, the *VANGL1*, *PCSK7*, and *ANXA3* genes showed the highest expression levels in most CRC samples.

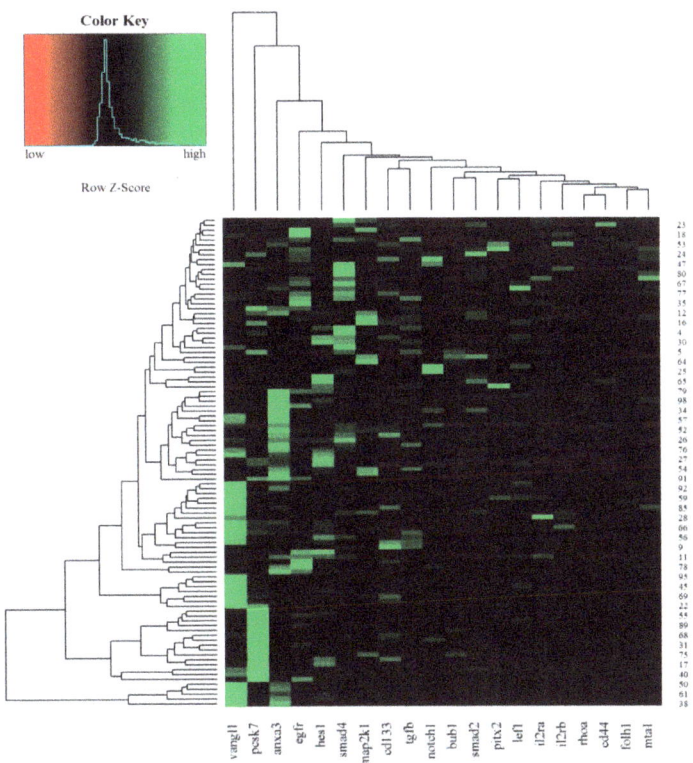

Figure 5. Heat maps of real-time RT-qPCR data representing gene expression variations of the 20 analyzed transcripts in FFPE CRC samples. Green indicates upregulation, and red indicates downregulation.

3.4. ROC Analysis

The predictive performance of the 20-gene signature was assessed by computing the AUC value of the ROC curve. A logistic regression model was built based on the comparison of tumor samples ($n = 100$) in relation to the following study patient characteristics: stage I–II vs. III–IV and presence vs. absence of LNM. We selected two panels including 5 and 10 genes based on the genes that had the highest AUC and showed a more effective role in CRC progression. One panel included 5 genes (*VANGL1*, *IL2RA*, *SMAD2*, *RHOA1*, and *HES*), and the other 10 genes (previous 5 plus *MTA1*, *CD133*, *FOLH1*, *NOTCH1*, and *TGF-ß*). The total number of genes (i.e., 20-gene panel) was also analyzed.

Figure 6 summarizes the performances of the study gene panels for the prediction of stage in the patient cohort, with the 20-gene panel achieving the highest performance. The AUC value for the 5-gene panel was 68.39%, along with 95% CI, 57.81%–78.97%; 67.30% sensitivity; and 66.66% specificity (Figure 6A); for the 10-gene panel, the AUC was 71.67% (95% CI, 61.51%–81.84%; sensitivity, 61.53%; and specificity, 72.91%) (Figure 6B). The analysis of the total 20 genes resulted in AUC = 78.85% (95% CI, 69.94%–87.75%; sensitivity, 75%; and specificity, 77.08%) (Figure 6C). In Figure 6D, the AUCs of 20-, 10-, and 5-gene panels in relation to stage are reported. When all the three AUCs (5-/10-/total-gene panels) were compared together, these results showed a trend towards significance ($p = 0.055$). When the AUC of the total number of genes was compared with that of the 5 genes, the difference was highly significant ($p = 0.02$). A statistical trend was observed between the AUC of the total panel and that of the 10-gene panel ($p = 0.08$), while no significant difference between the AUC of the 10-gene panel and that of the 5-gene panel was noted ($p = 0.34$).

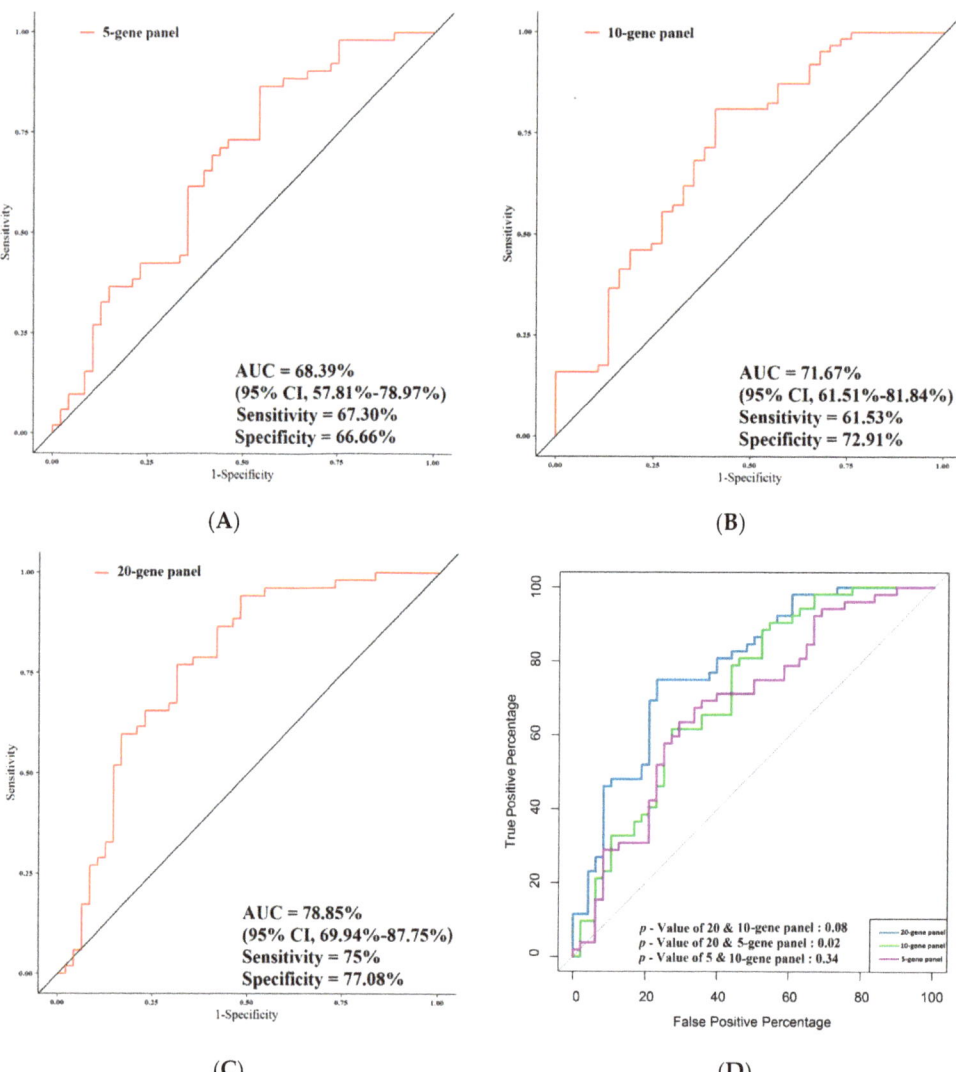

Figure 6. Comparison of the predictive performance by receiver operating characteristic (ROC) curve analysis for stage. (**A**) The AUC assessment of the logit(*p*) value for the panel of 5 genes. (**B**) The AUC assessment of the logit(*p*) value for the panel of 10 genes. (**C**) The AUC assessment of the logit(*p*) value for the panel of total genes. (**D**) Comparison of the predictive performance for the panel of 5, 10, and 20 genes.

Figure 7 summarizes the performances of the study gene panels for the prediction of LNMs in CRC patients, and also in this case, the 20-gene panel achieved the highest performance. The AUC value was 70.19% (95% CI, 59.18%–81.02%; sensitivity, 84.12%; specificity, 57.86%) when the gene expression of the 5-gene panel was compared in relation to LNM and non-LNM CRC patients (Figure 7A). Comparison of the gene expression of the 10-gene panel in relation to LNM and non-LNM CRC patients resulted in AUC = 71.47%

(95% CI, 60.62%–82.32%; sensitivity, 80.95%; specificity, 59.45%) (Figure 7B). The AUC of the total genes in LNM vs. non-LNM CRC patients was the highest of the three AUCs obtained (i.e., 79.84% (95% CI, 70.38%–89.30%; sensitivity, 74.60%; specificity, 75.67%) (Figure 7C). As far as the association with LNMs was concerned, the comparison between all the AUCs together (5-/10-/total-gene panels) pointed out a nearly significant difference ($p = 0.05$). In particular, the AUC of the total-gene panel was significantly higher compared with that of the 5-gene panel ($p = 0.03$) in relation to LNM and non-LNM CRC patients (Figure 7D). A high statistical trend was observed between the AUC of the total gene panel and that of the 10-gene panel ($p = 0.06$), although no statistical difference was observed between the AUC of the 10-gene panel and that of the 5-gene panel ($p = 0.38$). We also analyzed the predictive performance of single genes according to stage and LNM (Tables S1 and S2). Data showed that the *VANGL1* gene was a significant predictor for LNMs with an AUC of 63.99 (95% CI, 52.41%–75.56%; sensitivity, 80.95%; specificity, 45.94%).

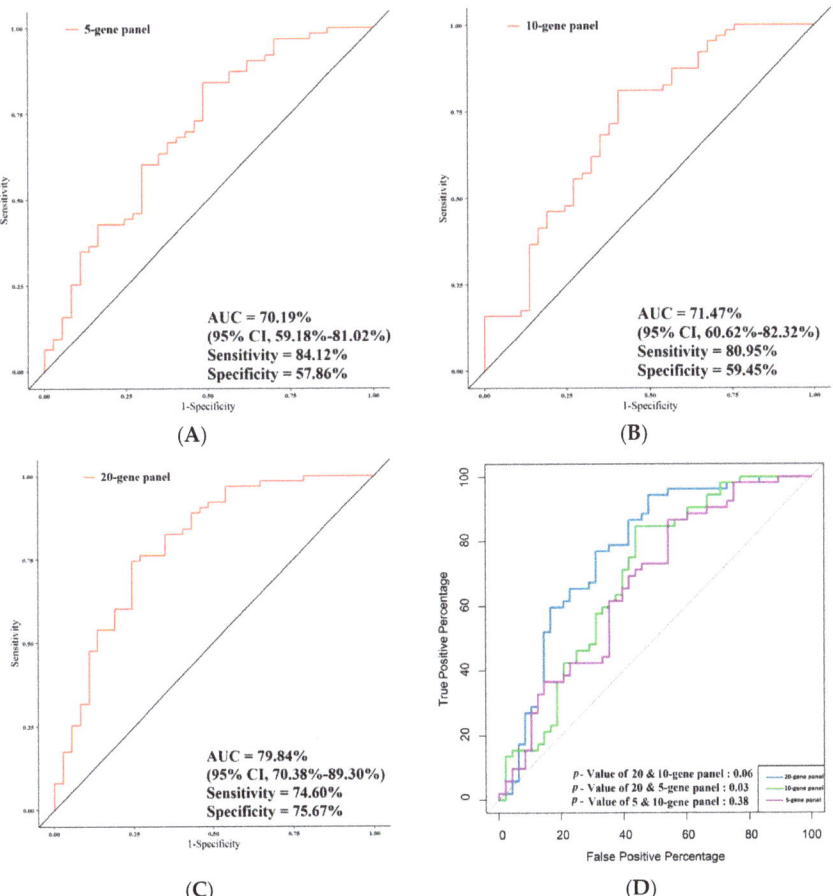

Figure 7. Comparison of the predictive performance by receiver operating characteristic (ROC) curve analysis for lymph node metastasis (LNMs). (**A**) The AUC assessment of the logit(*p*) value for the panel of 5 genes. (**B**) The AUC assessment of the logit(*p*) value for the panel of 10 genes. (**C**) The AUC assessment of the logit(*p*) value for the panel of total genes. (**D**) Comparison of the predictive performance for the panel of 5, 10, and 20 genes.

3.5. Correlation of Gene Expression with Overall Survival

All patients completed their follow-up by 20 December 2018 (median, 10.8 years, and range, 0.019–21 years). Patients whose tumors expressed higher levels of *NOTCH1* mRNA or lower levels of *IL2RB* mRNA showed a statistically significant prolonged OS compared with their respective counterparts ($p = 0.042$ and $p = 0.043$, respectively) (Figure 8). No other statistically significant correlation was found between OS and expression levels of the other study genes.

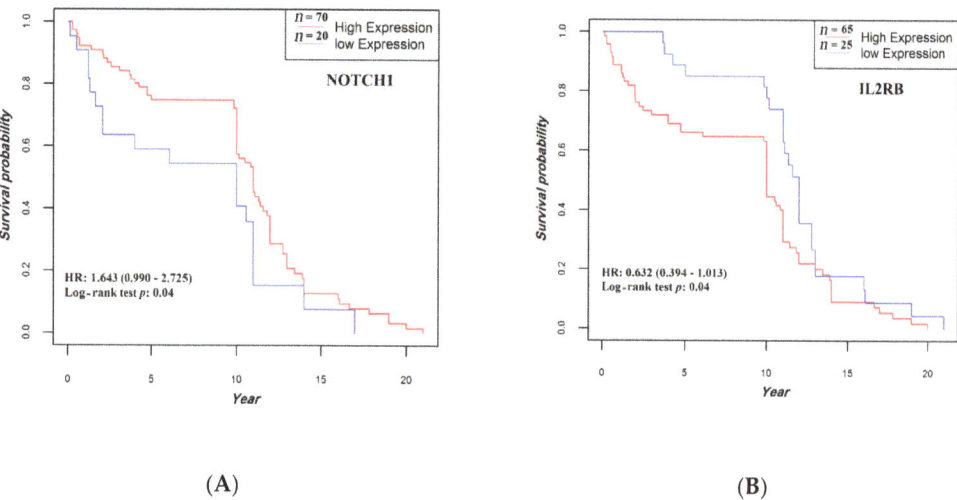

(A)   (B)

Figure 8. Association between *NOTCH1* (**A**) and *IL2RB* (**B**) expression and overall survival. The median follow-up was 10.8 (0.95LCL–0.95UCL; 10–11) years. HR, hazard ratio.

3.6. Immunohistochemistry Analysis

The protein expression levels of four genes that play a critical role in cancer development and progression was evaluated by using IHC. Twenty-five percent of CRC FFPE and normal matched tissues were used in this regard. In particular, we were interested in the evaluation of the expression levels of the products of *VANGL1*, *EGFR*, and *SMAD4* based on literature data and on the relationships we observed between the expression of their respective encoding genes and the clinical/pathological characteristics of the study CRC patients. The fourth protein we selected was LEF1. Although we did not find relationships between *LEF1* gene expression and the clinical/pathological parameters of CRC patients, we were interested in evaluating the potential role of LEF1 as an early biomarker of colorectal carcinogenesis since its activation by MYC has been associated with the activation of the WNT pathway signaling. The protein expression of VANGL1, EGFR, LEF1, and SMAD4 via their antibodies were examined. Results showed that VANGL1 and EGFR proteins were overexpressed (more than 50% of the stained cells in colon adenocarcinoma tissues compared with the normal tissues) (Figures 9 and 10). Additionally, immunohistochemical staining revealed a predominantly nuclear localization of SMAD4 and LEF1, and they showed higher expression in CRC tissues compared with normal colonic mucosa with more than 50% and 20% of the stained cells, respectively (Figures 10 and 11).

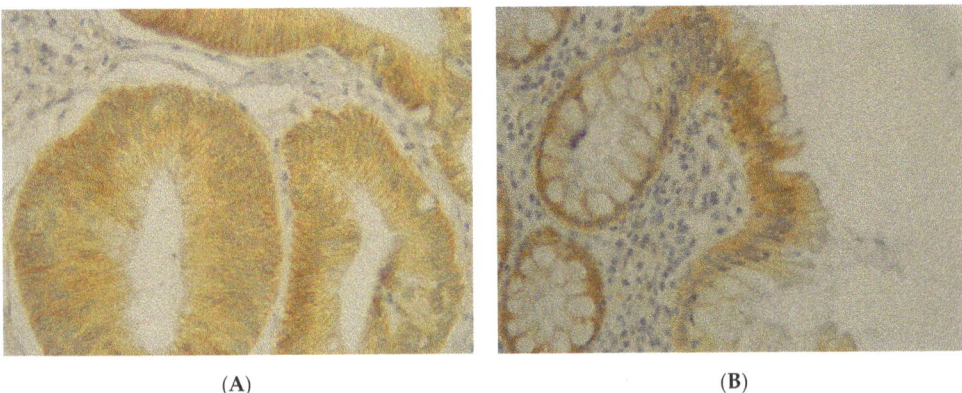

Figure 9. (**A**) Immunohistochemical staining of VANGL1 in colorectal adenocarcinoma with an intensity score of 3+ with more than 70% of the stained cells. (**B**) Immunohistochemical staining of VANGL1 in normal sample.

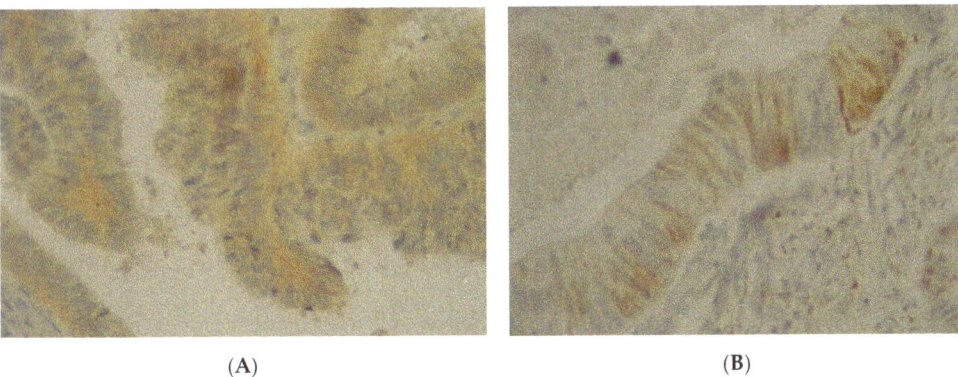

Figure 10. (**A**) Immunohistochemical staining of EGFR in colorectal adenocarcinoma with an intensity score of 2+ with more than 50% of the stained cells. (**B**) Immunohistochemical staining of LEF1 in colorectal adenocarcinoma with a positive expression of more than 20% of the stained cells.

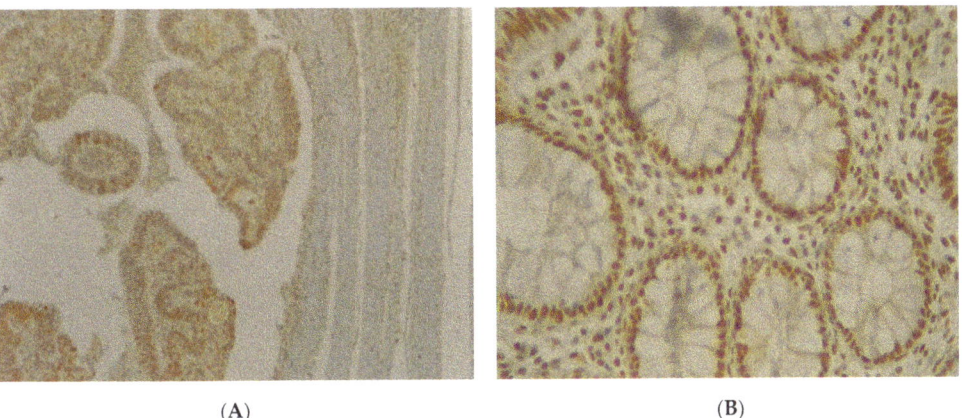

Figure 11. (**A**) Immunohistochemical staining of SMAD4 in colorectal adenocarcinoma with an intensity score of 2+ with more than 50% of the stained cells. (**B**) Immunohistochemical staining of SMAD4 in normal sample.

4. Discussion

The prediction of CRC progression risk and the identification of novel biomarkers predictive of this risk could represent a relevant advancement [6]. In this study, we evaluated the expression levels of several genes that are involved in LNM and malignant transitions in CRC tissues via RT-qPCR and IHC methods.

Previous investigations showed a high tumor expression level of the *VANGL-1* gene in CRC patients compared with normal tissues [21–24]. Additionally, *VANGL1* gene expression levels have been suggested to play a critical role in CRC progression and to be notably related to tumor stages and LNM [21–24]. These findings are in substantial agreement with our results. Lee and et al. showed that *VANGL1* gene knockdown can decrease the mRNA expression level of *CYKLIND1*, *COX2*, *MMP3*, and *ERK1/2* and reduce tumor growth and invasion. In addition, they found that a high expression level of the *VANGL1* gene was associated with the overexpression of *AP-1* target genes, which have an important role in MAPK signaling in CRC [22]. Oh et al. indicated that *VANGL1* silencing reduced vascular endothelial growth factor A (VEGF-A) and hypoxia-inducible factor 1-alpha (HIF1A). They suggested that the *VANGL1* gene can increase angiogenesis and CRC malignancy [21]. Additionally, our past investigations showed that angiogenesis and the angiogenic factors *VEGF-A* and *HIFA* play an important role in CRC initiation and progression [25–27]. Thus, it seems that the *VANGL1* gene may interact with VEGF-A and HIF1A signaling and enhance tumor malignancy.

In this study, we showed that the *VANGL1* gene was an independent prognostic biomarker for CRC patients. Taken together, these results indicate that the *VANGL1* gene may have a key role in the regulation of several genes, including those involved in angiogenesis. Thus, *VANGL1* could be suggested as a potential biomarker for the prediction of tumor malignancy and targeted therapy in CRC.

$TGF-\beta$ has been suggested to be a tumor suppressor gene able to stop the cell cycle at early stages of tumor, and SMAD proteins, being transcriptional mediators of $TGF-\beta$ signaling, play a critical role in it [28]. In particular, *SMAD2* is located at 18q21 and plays a role as a tumor suppressor gene [29–31]. As a result of the loss of heterozygosity (LOH) in the 18q21 region, *SMAD2* gene expression is reduced in several cancers and increases cancer progression [31]. However, our findings showed a significant downregulation of *SMAD2* in well-differentiated tumors. Although this finding is substantial in contrast with most of the available data, the complexity of the mutational profile of *SMAD2* [32], its relationships with the other SMAD proteins [33], and the potential role of specific miRNAs on the regulation of *SMAD2* [34] could have contributed to this result.

SMAD4 that forms a heterotrimer with *SMAD2* and *SMAD3* to exert transcriptional activity plays a crucial role in carcinogenesis [35], and loss of the *SMAD4* gene occurs in about 30% of CRC [36]. It was reported that loss of *SMAD4* was significantly related to CRC progression and metastasis and occurred in late stages [29,37–40]. Previous studies revealed that in colon cancer, the activation of $TGF-\beta$ signaling induced ERK and P38 signaling and stimulated angiogenesis by *VEGF* upregulation when *SMAD4* was knocked down [36]. Our findings are in agreement with previous investigations [41,42] and indicate that the expression level of the *SMAD4* gene in stage III-IV CRC was lower than that in stage I-II, although this difference did not reach a statistically significant level.

We observed an upregulation of the $TGF-\beta$ gene in stage III-IV CRC samples, although these results were not statistically significant. According to these data, loss of the *SMAD4* gene and upregulation of $TGF-\beta$ may be associated with a more advanced tumor stage and can promote cancer initiation, progression, and metastasis [35].

The NOTCH signaling pathway activity has been reported in several cancers, such as CRC and hepatocarcinoma [43–46]. NOTCH signaling consists of several receptors (NOTCH1–4) and targets genes including the transcription factor *HES1* (HES family basic helix-loop-helix (bHLH) transcription factor 1) [43,47,48]. In addition, *HES1* has several functions, such as intestinal cell stability and apoptosis control [43,49]. Our study showed a downregulation of *NOTCH1* in stage III-IV CRC and a significant correlation between a high expression level of NOTCH1 and longer patient survival. This is in contrast with a previous study that reported an upregulation of NOTCH1 in advanced or metastatic CRC patients and a significant association between the upregulation of NOTCH1 and poor survival [43]. Moreover, we observed a significant overexpression of NOTCH1 levels in female patients.

In agreement with our findings, several studies demonstrated a significant overexpression of the *HES1* gene in CRC samples compared with a normal tissue [50–52]. Additionally, we found that the overexpression of the *HES1* gene in stage III-IV CRC was more marked than in stage I-II. This result is in agreement with past investigations [43,50,52]. Overall, our data, together with those of others, confirm that NOTCH signaling, especially *NOTCH1* and *HES1*, play a critical role in metastasis and invasion as well as in the activation of several other signaling pathways. The activation of *NOTCH1* is, in fact, able to induce *HES1* and to start cancer progression [53–56].

IL2RA and *IL2RB* bind interleukin 2, which is necessary for the stimulation of T-cell immune response, and act as signal transduction factors. A high level of *IL2*, *IL2RA*, and *IL2RB* gene expression and their relationships with tumor progression and malignancy have been previously reported [57]. However, in agreement with our results, Marshall et al. also found no significant association between *IL2RB* gene expression and cancer progression [58]. In the present investigation, we observed that a downregulation of *IL2RA* was significantly associated with CRC patients younger than 50 years.

ANXA3 plays a relevant role in tumor metastasis, invasion, and drug treatment resistance [59–62]. In a previous investigation, a blood-based biomarker panel, also including the *ANXA3* gene, able to stratify subjects according to their relative CRC risk in comparison with an average-risk population, was developed [58]. Similar to this study, a significant upregulation of *ANXA3* has been identified in CRC tissues compared with normal mucosa as well as in several other cancers, such as pancreas, breast, and lung cancers [63,64].

Several findings have shown that the suppression of *ANXA3* upregulation could inhibit cell proliferation and metastasis in CRC [65,66]. Thus, *ANXA3* could be considered a new potential prognostic biomarker and therapeutic target for CRC treatment [66,67]. Upregulation of the *ANXA3* gene and its correlation with gastric tumor size, stage, and LNMs were detected by Wang et al. [67] Moreover, these authors suggested that the overexpression of ANXA3 has a huge effect on gastric cancer malignancy, and it can be used as a novel prognostic biomarker and a suitable target for treatment [67]. Zhou et al. reported that high expression levels of ANXA3 were significantly correlated with breast tumor LNMs and tumor grade, suggesting ANXA3 as a biomarker for breast cancer prognosis [68]. In our study, a significant overexpression of the *ANXA3* gene in well-differentiated tumors compared with poorly differentiated tumors was instead observed. However, we also observed higher levels of *ANXA3* in tumors from patients with LNMs compared with tumors from patients without LNMs, although this difference did not reach statistical significance. Overall, we were only able to partially confirm the observations of other authors who suggested that the *ANXA3* gene may act as an oncogene and play a role in the transformation of a normal tissue into tumor, CRC invasion, and malignancy progression.

BUB1 acts as a checkpoint factor during cell mitosis and proliferation, and *PCSK7* plays a role in cellular multiplication, mortality, and adhesion. These two genes are involved in cancer metastasis and invasion [69–72]. In our study, we observed a downregulation of the *BUB1* gene in CRC samples compared with normal mucosa, but this difference was not statistically significant. Additionally, previous studies showed a downregulation of the *BUB1* gene in gastric cancer and in CRC [70,73]. Furthermore, in agreement with previous studies, we found an upregulation of *PCSK7* in CRC. On the other hand, Jaaks et al. realized a significant upregulation of the *PCSK7* gene in colon cancer and considered it a potential biomarker [72]. Taken together, it could be suggested that the low expression level of *BUB1* and the upregulation of *PCSK7* have a critical role in malignant transition through colorectal carcinogenesis.

EGFR is a transmembrane receptor that binds to EGF and stimulates cell growth in tissues. Overexpression of the *EGFR* gene has been observed in several cancers, including colorectal, lung, breast, and bladder [74]. It has been reported that the *EGFR* gene may play a role in CRC development [75] since its expression increases with malignant transformation from normal colonic mucosa to metastatic CRC [75,76]. Previous studies, in fact, showed that *EGFR* gene overexpression was significantly related to tumor stages, metastasis, and well-differentiated tumors [75,77]. Although we found a higher expression of *EGFR* in tumor tissues compared with normal tissues, as well as in the right colon compared with the left colon, we did not find correlations between tumor *EGFR* gene expression and clinicopathological features. However, our observations substantially confirm the role of EGFR in CRC progression.

5. Conclusions

In conclusion, the main results of this study highlight that the expression of the tumor *VANGL1* gene is an independent prognostic biomarker and could be considered a potential predictor for detecting malignancy risk in CRC patients. Additionally, LNMs were highly predicted by the 20-gene panels. However, validation studies including a higher number of patients are required.

Supplementary Materials: The following are available online at https://www.mdpi.com/2075-4426/11/2/126/s1, Table S1: Logistic Regression Test of the 20 Genes (Analysis–Metastasis); Table S2: Logistic Regression Test of the 20 Genes (Analysis–Stage).

Author Contributions: Conceptualization, N.P. and E.N.M.; data curation, S.N., E.M., and E.N.M.; formal analysis, M.O.; funding acquisition, H.A.A.; investigation, E.N.M.; methodology, N.P., A.M., K.B., F.A., and E.N.M.; project administration, E.N.M.; resources, H.A.A. and M.R.Z.; software, N.P.; supervision, E.N.M.; validation, Z.P.; visualization, K.N.; writing—original draft, N.P., Z.P., and E.N.M.; writing—review and editing, N.P., S.N., Z.P., E.M., and E.N.M. All authors have read and agreed to the published version of the manuscript.

Funding: This project was completely supported and funded by the Gastroenterology and Liver Diseases Research Center, Research Institute for Gastroenterology and Liver Diseases, Shahid Beheshti University of Medical Sciences, with Grant Nos. 858 and 988, and the Medical Ethical Committee of the RCGLD, with Ethics No. IR.SBMU.RIGLD.REC.1396.947.

Institutional Review Board Statement: This study was approved by the ethical committee (Ethics No. IR.SBMU.RIGLD.REC.1396.947) of the Research Institute for Gastroenterology and Liver Disease, Shahid Beheshti University of Medical Sciences, Tehran, Iran.

Informed Consent Statement: Informed consent was obtained from all subjects involved in the study.

Data Availability Statement: The data presented in this study are available on request from the corresponding author.

Acknowledgments: The authors would like to thank all the staff of the Cancer Department in the Research Institute for Gastroenterology and Liver Diseases, Shahid Beheshti University of Medical Sciences, Tehran, Iran.

Conflicts of Interest: The authors declare no potential conflicts of interest with respect to the research, authorship, and/or publication of this article.

References

1. Ueda, Y.; Yasuda, K.; Inomata, M.; Shiraishi, N.; Yokoyama, S.; Kitano, S. Biological predictors of survival in stage II colorectal cancer. *Mol. Clin. Oncol.* **2013**, *1*, 643–648. [CrossRef]
2. Ong, M.L.H.; Schofield, J.B. Assessment of lymph node involvement in colorectal cancer. *World J. Gastrointest. Surg.* **2016**, *8*, 179–192. [CrossRef]
3. Benson, A.B.; Venook, A.P.; Al-Hawary, M.M.; Arain, M.A.; Chen, Y.-J.; Ciombor, K.K.; Cohen, S.; Cooper, H.S.; Deming, D.; Farkas, L.; et al. Colon Cancer, Version 2.2.2021, NCCN Clinical Practice Guidelines in Oncology. Available online: www.nccn.org/professionals/physician_gls/pdf/colon/pdf (accessed on 1 February 2021).

4. Schell, M.J.; Yang, M.; Missiaglia, E.; Delorenzi, M.; Soneson, C.; Yue, B.; Nebozhyn, M.V.; Loboda, A.; Bloom, G.; Yeatman, T.J. A Composite Gene Expression Signature Optimizes Prediction of Colorectal Cancer Metastasis and Outcome. *Clin. Cancer Res.* **2016**, *22*, 734–745. [CrossRef] [PubMed]
5. Kim, H.J.; Choi, G. Clinical Implications of Lymph Node Metastasis in Colorectal Cancer: Current Status and Future Perspectives. *Ann. Coloproctol.* **2019**, *35*, 109–117. [CrossRef]
6. Peyravian, N.; Larki, P.; Gharib, E.; Sadeghi, H.; Anaraki, F.; Young, C.; McClellan, J.; Bonab, M.A.; Asadzadeh-Aghdaei, H.; Zali, M.R. The Application of Gene Expression Profiling in Predictions of Occult Lymph Node Metastasis in Colorectal Cancer Patients. *Biomedicines* **2018**, *6*, 27. [CrossRef]
7. Nicastri, D.G.; Doucette, J.T.; Godfrey, T.E.; Hughes, S.J. Is Occult Lymph Node Disease in Colorectal Cancer Patients Clinically Significant? *J. Mol. Diagn.* **2007**, *9*, 563–571. [CrossRef] [PubMed]
8. Amin, M.B.; Greene, F.L.; Edge, S.B.; Compton, C.C.; Gershenwald, J.E.; Brookland, R.K.; Meyer, L.; Gress, D.M.; Byrd, D.R.; Winchester, D.P. The Eighth Edition AJCC Cancer Staging Manual: Continuing to build a bridge from a population-based to a more "personalized" approach to cancer staging. *Cancer J. Clin.* **2017**, *67*, 93–99. [CrossRef]
9. Mojarad, E.N.; Kuppen, P.J.; Aghdaei, H.A.; Zali, M.R. The CpG island methylator phenotype (CIMP) in colorectal cancer. *Gastroenterol. Hepatol. Bed Bench* **2013**, *6*, 120–128.
10. Esfahani, A.T.; Seyedna, S.Y.; Nazemalhosseini-Mojarad, E.; Majd, A.; Aghdaei, H.A. MSI-L/EMAST is a predictive biomarker for metastasis in colorectal cancer patients. *J. Cell. Physiol.* **2019**, *234*, 13128–13136. [CrossRef]
11. Nazemalhosseini-Mojarad, E.; Mohammadpour, S.; Esafahani, A.T.; Gharib, E.; Larki, P.; Moradi, A.; Porhoseingholi, M.A.; Aghdaei, H.A.; Kuppen, P.J.K.; Zali, M.R. Intratumoral infiltrating lymphocytes correlate with improved survival in colorectal cancer patients: Independent of oncogenetic features. *J. Cell. Physiol.* **2019**, *234*, 4768–4777. [CrossRef] [PubMed]
12. Petrelli, F.; Ghidini, M.; Cabiddu, M.; Pezzica, E.; Corti, D.; Turati, L.; Costanzo, A.; Varricchio, A.; Ghidini, A.; Barni, S.; et al. Microsatellite Instability and Survival in Stage II Colorectal Cancer: A Systematic Review and Meta-analysis. *Anticancer Res.* **2019**, *39*, 6431–6441. [CrossRef] [PubMed]
13. Yan, X.; Wan, H.; Hao, X.; Lan, T.; Li, W.; Xu, L.; Yuan, K.; Wu, H. Importance of gene expression signatures in pancreatic cancer prognosis and the establishment of a prediction model. *Cancer Manag. Res.* **2018**, *11*, 273–283. [CrossRef]
14. Angadi, P.; Kale, A. Tumor budding is a potential histopathological marker in the prognosis of oral squamous cell carcinoma: Current status and future prospects. *J. Oral Maxillofac. Pathol.* **2019**, *23*, 318. [CrossRef] [PubMed]
15. Dihge, L.; Vallon-Christersson, J.; Hegardt, C.; Saal, L.H.; Häkkinen, J.; Larsson, C.; Ehinger, A.; Loman, N.; Malmberg, M.; Bendahl, P.-O.; et al. Prediction of Lymph Node Metastasis in Breast Cancer by Gene Expression and Clinicopathological Models: Development and Validation within a Population-Based Cohort. *Clin. Cancer Res.* **2019**, *25*, 6368–6381. [CrossRef] [PubMed]
16. Meeh, P.F.; Farrell, C.L.; Croshaw, R.; Crimm, H.; Miller, S.K.; Oroian, D.; Kowli, S.; Zhu, J.; Carver, W.; Wu, W.; et al. A Gene Expression Classifier of Node-Positive Colorectal Cancer. *Neoplasia* **2009**, *11*, 1074-IN12. [CrossRef]
17. Dai, W.; Li, Y.; Mo, S.; Feng, Y.; Zhang, L.; Xu, Y.; Li, Q.; Cai, G. A robust gene signature for the prediction of early relapse in stage I-III colon cancer. *Mol. Oncol.* **2018**, *12*, 463–475. [CrossRef]
18. Chu, C.-M.; Yao, C.-T.; Chang, Y.-T.; Chou, H.-L.; Chou, Y.-C.; Chen, K.-H.; Terng, H.-J.; Huang, C.-S.; Lee, C.-C.; Su, S.-L.; et al. Gene Expression Profiling of Colorectal Tumors and Normal Mucosa by Microarrays Meta-Analysis Using Prediction Analysis of Microarray, Artificial Neural Network, Classification, and Regression Trees. *Dis. Markers* **2014**, *2014*, 1–11. [CrossRef]
19. Gutiérrez, M.L.; Corchete-Sánchez, L.A.; Sarasquete, M.E.; Abad, M.D.M.; Bengoechea, O.; Fermiñán, E.; Anduaga, M.F.; Del Carmen, S.; Iglesias, M.; Esteban, C.; et al. Prognostic impact of a novel gene expression profile classifier for the discrimination between metastatic and non-metastatic primary colorectal cancer tumors. *Oncotarget* **2017**, *8*, 107685–107700. [CrossRef] [PubMed]
20. Kleivi, K.; Lind, G.E.; Diep, C.B.; Meling, G.I.; Brandal, L.T.; Nesland, J.M.; Myklebost, O.; Rognum, T.O.; Giercksky, K.-E.; Skotheim, R.I.; et al. Gene expression profiles of primary colorectal carcinomas, liver metastases, and carcinomatoses. *Mol. Cancer* **2007**, *6*, 2. [CrossRef]
21. Oh, H.-H.; Park, K.-J.; Kim, N.; Park, S.-Y.; Park, Y.-L.; Oak, C.-Y.; Myung, D.S.; Cho, S.-B.; Lee, W.-S.; Kim, K.-K.; et al. Impact of KITENIN on tumor angiogenesis and lymphangiogenesis in colorectal cancer. *Oncol. Rep.* **2015**, *35*, 253–260. [CrossRef] [PubMed]
22. Lee, S.; Song, Y.-A.; Park, Y.-L.; Cho, S.-B.; Lee, W.-S.; Lee, J.-H.; Chung, I.-J.; Kim, K.-K.; Rew, J.-S.; Joo, H.-H.O.A.Y.-E. Expression of KITENIN in human colorectal cancer and its relation to tumor behavior and progression. *Pathol. Int.* **2011**, *61*, 210–220. [CrossRef]
23. Bae, J.A.; Kho, D.H.; Sun, E.G.; Ko, Y.-S.; Yoon, S.; Lee, K.H.; Ahn, K.Y.; Lee, K.-H.; Joo, H.-H.O.A.Y.-E.; Chung, I.-J.; et al. Elevated Coexpression of KITENIN and the ErbB4 CYT-2 Isoform Promotes the Transition from Colon Adenoma to Carcinoma Following APC loss. *Clin. Cancer Res.* **2016**, *22*, 1284–1294. [CrossRef]
24. Sun, E.G.; Lee, K.H.; Ko, Y.-S.; Choi, H.J.; Yang, J.-I.; Lee, K.-H.; Chung, I.-J.; Paek, Y.-W.; Kim, H.; Bae, J.A.; et al. KITENIN functions as a fine regulator of ErbB4 expression level in colorectal cancer via protection of ErbB4 from E3-ligase Nrdp1-mediated degradation. *Mol. Carcinog.* **2016**, *56*, 1068–1081. [CrossRef] [PubMed]
25. Pezeshkian, Z.; Forouzesh, F.; Peyravian, N.; Yaghoob-Taleghani, M.; Asadzadeh-Aghdaei, H.; Zali, M.; Nazemalhosseini-Mojarad, E. Clinicopatho-logical correlations of VEGF-A and MMP-7 genes expression in different types of colorectal adenoma polyps. *WCRJ* **2017**, *4*, e978.
26. Aghdaei, H.A.; Pezeshkian, Z.; Abdollahpour-Alitappeh, M.; Nazemalhosseini-Mojarad, E.; Zali, M.R. The Role of Angiogenesis in Colorectal Polyps and Cancer, a Review. *Med. Lab. J.* **2018**, *12*, 1–6. [CrossRef]

27. Khatibi, S.; Nazemalhosseini Mojarad, E.; Forouzesh, F.; Pezeshkian, Z.; Asadzadeh Aghdaei, H.; Zali, M.R. HIF-1 alpha gene expression is not a suitable biomarker for evaluating malignancy risk in colorectal polyps. *WCRJ* **2018**, *5*, e1128.
28. Massagué, J.; Blain, S.W.; Lo, R.S. TGFβ Signaling in Growth Control, Cancer, and Heritable Disorders. *Cell* **2000**, *103*, 295–309. [CrossRef]
29. Samanta, D. Alterations in the Smad pathway in human cancers. *Front. Biosci.* **2012**, *17*, 1281–1293. [CrossRef] [PubMed]
30. Fukushima, T.; Mashiko, M.; Takita, K.; Otake, T.; Endo, Y.; Sekikawa, K.; Takenoshita, S. Mutational analysis of TGF-β type II receptor, Smad2, Smad3, Smad4, Smad6 and Smad7 genes in colorectal cancer. *J. Exp. Clin. Cancer. Res.* **2003**, *22*, 315–320. [PubMed]
31. Tian, F.; Byfield, S.D.; Parks, W.T.; Yoo, S.; Felici, A.; Tang, B.; Piek, E.; Wakefield, L.M.; Roberts, A.B. Reduction in Smad2/3 signaling enhances tumorigenesis but suppresses metastasis of breast cancer cell lines. *Cancer. Res.* **2003**, *63*, 8284–8292. [PubMed]
32. Fleming, N.I.; Jorissen, R.N.; Mouradov, D.; Christie, M.; Sakthianandeswaren, A.; Palmieri, M.; Day, F.; Li, S.; Tsui, C.; Lipton, L.; et al. SMAD2, SMAD3 and SMAD4 Mutations in Colorectal Cancer. *Cancer Res.* **2013**, *73*, 725–735. [CrossRef]
33. Koveitypour, Z.; Panahi, F.; Vakilian, M.; Peymani, M.; Forootan, F.S.; Esfahani, M.H.N.; Ghaedi, K. Signaling pathways involved in colorectal cancer progression. *Cell Biosci.* **2019**, *9*, 1–14. [CrossRef]
34. Bao, Y.; Chen, Z.; Guo, Y.; Feng, Y.; Li, Z.; Han, W.; Wang, J.; Zhao, W.; Jiao, Y.; Li, K.; et al. Tumor Suppressor MicroRNA-27a in Colorectal Carcinogenesis and Progression by Targeting SGPP1 and Smad2. *PLoS ONE* **2014**, *9*, e105991. [CrossRef]
35. Zhao, M.; Mishra, L.; Deng, C.X. The role of TGF-β/SMAD4 signaling in cancer. *Int. J. Biol. Sci.* **2018**, *14*, 111–123. [CrossRef] [PubMed]
36. Papageorgis, P.; Cheng, K.H.; Ozturk, S.; Gong, Y.; Lambert, A.; Mostafavi Abdolmaleky, H.; Zhou, J.-R.; Thiagalingam, S. Smad4 Inactivation Pro-motes Malignancy and Drug Resistance of Colon Cancer. *Cancer. Res.* **2011**, *71*, 998–1008. [CrossRef]
37. Maitra, A.; Molberg, K.; Albores-Saavedra, J.; Lindberg, G. Loss of Dpc4 Expression in Colonic Adenocarcinomas Correlates with the Presence of Metastatic Disease. *Am. J. Pathol.* **2000**, *157*, 1105–1111. [CrossRef]
38. Miyaki, M.; Iijima, T.; Konishi, M.; Sakai, K.; Ishii, A.; Yasuno, M.; Hishima, T.; Koike, M.; Shitara, N.; Iwama, T.; et al. Higher frequency of Smad4 gene mutation in human colorectal cancer with distant metastasis. *Oncogene* **1999**, *18*, 3098–3103. [CrossRef] [PubMed]
39. Kitamura, T.; Kometani, K.; Hashida, H.; Matsunaga, A.; Miyoshi, H.; Hosogi, H.; Aoki, M.; Oshima, M.; Hattori, M.; Takabayashi, A.; et al. SMAD4-deficient intestinal tumors recruit CCR1+ myeloid cells that promote invasion. *Nat. Genet.* **2007**, *39*, 467–475. [CrossRef]
40. Inamoto, S.; Itatani, Y.; Yamamoto, T.; Minamiguchi, S.; Hirai, H.; Iwamoto, M.; Hasegawa, S.; Taketo, M.M.; Sakai, Y.; Kawada, K. Loss of SMAD4 Promotes Colorectal Cancer Progression by Accumulation of Myeloid-Derived Suppressor Cells through the CCL15–CCR1 Chemokine Axis. *Clin. Cancer Res.* **2016**, *22*, 492–501. [CrossRef]
41. Calon, A.; Lonardo, E.; Berenguer-Llergo, A.; Espinet, E.; Hernando-Momblona, X.; Iglesias, M.; Sevillano, M.; Palomo-Ponce, S.; Tauriello, D.V.F.; Byrom, D.; et al. Stromal gene expression defines poor-prognosis subtypes in colorectal cancer. *Nat. Genet.* **2015**, *47*, 320–329. [CrossRef] [PubMed]
42. Li, H.; Zhang, Z.; Chen, L.; Sun, X.; Zhao, Y.; Guo, Q.; Zhu, S.; Li, P.; Min, L.; Zhang, S. Cytoplasmic Asporin promotes cell migration by regulating TGF-β/Smad2/3 pathway and indicates a poor prognosis in colorectal cancer. *Cell Death Dis.* **2019**, *10*, 1–14. [CrossRef]
43. Huang, R.; Tang, Q.; You, Q.; Liu, Z.; Wang, G.; Chen, Y.; Sun, Y.; Muhammad, S.; Wang, X. Disparity Expression of Notch1 in Benign and Malignant Colorectal Diseases. *PLoS ONE* **2013**, *8*, e81005. [CrossRef]
44. Androutsellis-Theotokis, A.; Leker, R.R.; Soldner, F.; Hoeppner, D.J.; Ravin, R.; Poser, S.W.; Rueger, M.A.; Bae, S.-K.; Kittappa, R.; McKay, R.D.G. Notch signalling regulates stem cell numbers in vitro and in vivo. *Nat. Cell Biol.* **2006**, *442*, 823–826. [CrossRef]
45. Okamoto, R.; Tsuchiya, K.; Nemoto, Y.; Akiyama, J.; Nakamura, T.; Kanai, T.; Watanabe, M. Requirement of Notch activation during regeneration of the intestinal epithelia. *Am. J. Physiol. Liver Physiol.* **2009**, *296*, 23–35. [CrossRef]
46. Chen, X.; Stoeck, A.; Lee, S.J.; Shih, I.-M.; Wang, M.M.; Wang, T.-L. Jagged1 Expression Regulated by Notch3 and Wnt/β-catenin Signaling Pathways in Ovarian Cancer. *Oncotarget* **2010**, *1*, 210–218. [CrossRef] [PubMed]
47. Wang, H.; Zang, C.; Liu, X.S.; Aster, J.C. The role of Notch receptors in transcriptional Regulation. *J. Cell Physiol.* **2015**, *230*, 982–988. [CrossRef]
48. Lutgens, M.W.M.D.; Vleggaar, F.P.; Schipper, M.E.I.; Stokkers, P.C.F.; Van Der Woude, C.J.; Hommes, D.W.; De Jong, D.J.; Dijkstra, G.; Van Bodegraven, A.A.; Oldenburg, B.; et al. High frequency of early colorectal cancer in inflammatory bowel disease. *Gut* **2008**, *57*, 1246–1251. [CrossRef]
49. Kageyama, R.; Ohtsuka, T.; Kobayashi, T. The Hes gene family: Repressors and oscillators that orchestrate embryogenesis. *Development* **2007**, *134*, 1243–1251. [CrossRef] [PubMed]
50. Yuan, R.; Ke, J.; Sun, L.; He, Z.; Zou, Y.; He, X.; Chen, Y.; Wu, X.; Cai, Z.; Wang, L.; et al. HES1 promotes metastasis and predicts poor survival in patients with colorectal cancer. *Clin. Exp. Metastasis* **2015**, *32*, 169–179. [CrossRef]
51. Egan, S.E.; Reedijk, M.; Odorcic, S.; Zhang, H.; Chetty, R.; Tennert, C.; Dickson, B.C.; Lockwood, G.; Gallinger, S. Activation of Notch signaling in human colon adenocarcinoma. *Int. J. Oncol.* **1992**, *33*, 1223–1229. [CrossRef] [PubMed]
52. Candy, P.A.; Phillips, M.R.; Redfern, A.D.; Colley, S.M.; Davidson, J.A.; Stuart, L.M.; A. Wood, B.; Zeps, N.; Leedman, P.J. Notch-induced transcription factors are predictive of survival and 5-fluorouracil response in colorectal cancer patients. *Br. J. Cancer* **2013**, *109*, 1023–1030. [CrossRef] [PubMed]

53. Rajendran, D.T.; Subramaniyan, B.; Mathan, G. Role of Notch Signaling in Colorectal Cancer. *Role Transcr. Factors Gastrointest. Malig.* **2017**, 307–314. [CrossRef]
54. Zhang, P.; Yang, Y.; Zweidler-McKay, P.A.; Hughes, D.P. Critical Role of Notch Signaling in Osteosarcoma Invasion and Metastasis. *Clin. Cancer Res.* **2008**, *14*, 2962–2969. [CrossRef] [PubMed]
55. Wang, Z.; Banerjee, S.; Li, Y.; Rahman, K.M.W.; Zhang, Y.-X.; Sarkar, F.H. Down-regulation of Notch-1 Inhibits Invasion by Inactivation of Nuclear Factor-κB, Vascular Endothelial Growth Factor, and Matrix Metalloproteinase-9 in Pancreatic Cancer Cells. *Cancer Res.* **2006**, *66*, 2778–2784. [CrossRef] [PubMed]
56. Balint, K.; Xiao, M.; Pinnix, C.C.; Soma, A.; Veres, I.; Juhasz, I.; Brown, E.J.; Capobianco, A.J.; Herlyn, M.; Liu, Z.-J. Activation of Notch1 signaling is required for -catenin-mediated human primary melanoma progression. *J. Clin. Investig.* **2005**, *115*, 3166–3176. [CrossRef] [PubMed]
57. García-Tuñnón, I.; Ricote, M.; Ruiz, A.; Fraile, B.; Paniagua, R.; Royuela, M. Interleukin-2 and its receptor complex (α, β and γ chains) in in situ and infiltrative human breast cancer: An immunohistochemical comparative study. *Breast Cancer Res.* **2003**, *6*, R1–R7. [CrossRef] [PubMed]
58. Marshall, K.W.; Mohr, S.; El Khettabi, F.; Nossova, N.; Chao, S.; Bao, W.; Ma, J.; Li, X.-J.; Liew, C.-C. A blood-based biomarker panel for stratifying current risk for colorectal cancer. *Int. J. Cancer* **2009**, *126*, 1177–1186. [CrossRef]
59. Draeger, A.; Monastyrskaya, K.; Babiychuk, E.B. Plasma membrane repair and cellular damage control: The annexin survival kit. *Biochem Pharmacol.* **2011**, *81*, 703–712. [CrossRef]
60. Park, J.E.; Lee, D.H.; Lee, J.A.; Park, S.G.; Kim, N.-S.; Park, B.C.; Cho, S. Annexin A3 is a potential angiogenic mediator. *Biochem. Biophys. Res. Commun.* **2005**, *337*, 1283–1287. [CrossRef]
61. Harashima, M.; Harada, K.; Ito, Y.; Hyuga, M.; Seki, T.; Ariga, T.; Yamaguchi, T.; Niimi, S. Annexin A3 Expression Increases in Hepatocytes and is Regulated by Hepatocyte Growth Factor in Rat Liver Regeneration. *J. Biochem.* **2007**, *143*, 537–545. [CrossRef]
62. Yan, X.; Yin, J.; Yao, H.; Mao, N.; Yang, Y.; Pan, L. Increased Expression of Annexin A3 Is a Mechanism of Platinum Re-sistance in Ovarian Cancer. *Cancer. Res.* **2010**, *70*, 1616–1624. [CrossRef]
63. Wu, N.; Sun, M.-Z.; Guo, C.; Hou, Z.; Sun, M.-Z. The role of annexin A3 playing in cancers. *Clin. Transl. Oncol.* **2013**, *15*, 106–110. [CrossRef]
64. Zhou, T.; Liu, S.; Yang, L.; Ju, Y.; Li, C. The expression of ANXA3 and its relationship with the occurrence and development of breast cancer. *J. BUON* **2018**, *23*, 713–719. [PubMed]
65. Bai, Z.; Wang, J.; Wang, T.; Li, Y.; Zhao, X.; Wu, G.; Yang, Y.; Deng, W.; Zhang, Z. The MiR-495/Annexin A3/P53 Axis Inhibits the Invasion and EMT of Colorectal Cancer Cells. *Cell. Physiol. Biochem.* **2017**, *44*, 1882–1895. [CrossRef]
66. Yang, L.; Men, W.-L.; Yan, K.-M.; Tie, J.; Nie, Y.-Z.; Xiao, H.-J. MiR-340-5p is a potential prognostic indicator of colorectal cancer and modulates ANXA3. *Eur. Rev. Med. Pharmacol. Sci.* **2018**, *22*, 4837–4845. [PubMed]
67. Wang, K.; Li, J. Overexpression of ANXA3 is an independent prognostic indicator in gastric cancer and its depletion suppresses cell proliferation and tumor growth. *Oncotarget* **2016**, *7*, 86972–86984. [CrossRef]
68. Zhou, T.; Li, Y.; Yang, L.; Tang, T.; Zhang, L.; Shi, J. Annexin A3 as a Prognostic Biomarker for Breast Cancer: A Retrospective Study. *BioMed Res. Int.* **2017**, *2017*, 1–7. [CrossRef] [PubMed]
69. Shigeishi, H.; Oue, N.; Kuniyasu, H.; Wakikawa, A.; Yokozaki, H.; Ishikawa, T.; Yasui, W. Expression of Bub1 Gene Correlates with Tumor Proliferating Activity in Human Gastric Carcinomas. *Pathobiology* **2001**, *69*, 24–29. [CrossRef] [PubMed]
70. Stahl, D.; Braun, M.; Gentles, A.J.; Lingohr, P.; Walter, A.; Kristiansen, G.; Gütgemann, I. Low BUB1 expression is an adverse prognostic marker in gastric adenocarcinoma. *Oncotarget* **2017**, *8*, 76329–76339. [CrossRef]
71. Rounseville, M.P.; Davis, T.P. Prohormone convertase and autocrine growth factor mRNAs are coexpressed in small cell lung carcinoma. *J. Mol. Endocrinol.* **2000**, *25*, 121–128. [CrossRef]
72. Jaaks, P.; Bernasconi, M. The proprotein convertase furin in tumour progression. *Int. J. Cancer* **2017**, *141*, 654–663. [CrossRef] [PubMed]
73. Shichiri, M.; Yoshinaga, K.; Hisatomi, H.; Sugihara, K.; Hirata, Y. Genetic and epigenetic inactivation of mitotic checkpoint genes hBUB1 and hBUBR1 and their relationship to survival. *Cancer Res.* **2002**, *62*, 11782350.
74. Nicholson, R.; Gee, J.M.; Harper, M.E. EGFR and cancer prognosis. *Eur. J. Cancer* **2001**, *37* (Suppl. 4), 9–15. [CrossRef]
75. Repetto, L.; Gianni, W.; Aglianò, A.M.; Gazzaniga, P. Impact of EGFR expression on colorectal cancer patient prognosis and survival: A response. *Ann. Oncol.* **2005**, *16*, 1557. [CrossRef] [PubMed]
76. Goldstein, N.; Armin, M. Epidermal growth factor receptor immunohistochemical reactivity in patients with American Joint Committee on Cancer Stage IV colon adenocarcinoma: Implications for a standardized scoring system. *Cancer* **2001**, *92*, 1331–1346. [CrossRef]
77. McKay, J.A.; Murray, L.J.; Curran, S.; Ross, V.G.; Clark, C.; Murray, G.I.; Cassidy, J.; McLeod, H.L. Evaluation of the epidermal growth factor receptor (EGFR) in colorectal tumours and lymph node metastases. *Eur. J. Cancer* **2002**, *38*, 2258–2264. [CrossRef]

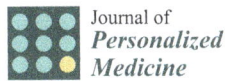

Article

Precision Medicine for the Management of Therapy Refractory Colorectal Cancer

Hossein Taghizadeh [1,2], Robert M. Mader [1,2], Leonhard Müllauer [2,3], Friedrich Erhart [4], Alexandra Kautzky-Willer [5] and Gerald W. Prager [1,2,*]

1. Department of Medicine I, Clinical Division of Oncology, Medical University of Vienna, 1090 Vienna, Austria; seyed.taghizadehwaghefi@meduniwien.ac.at (H.T.); robert.mader@meduniwien.ac.at (R.M.M.)
2. Comprehensive Cancer Center Vienna, 1090 Vienna, Austria; leonhard.muellauer@meduniwien.ac.at
3. Clinical Institute of Pathology, Medical University Vienna, 1090 Vienna, Austria
4. Department of Internal Medicine, Amstetten Region State Clinic, 3300 Amstetten, Austria; Friedrich.Erhart@amstetten.lknoe.at
5. Department of Medicine III, Gender Medicine Unit, Medical University of Vienna, 1090 Vienna, Austria; alexandra.kautzky-willer@meduniwien.ac.at
* Correspondence: gerald.prager@meduniwien.ac.at; Tel.: +43-1-40400-44500

Received: 14 October 2020; Accepted: 9 December 2020; Published: 11 December 2020

Abstract: In this analysis, we examined the efficacy, feasibility, and limitations of molecular-based targeted therapies in heavily pretreated metastatic colorectal cancer (mCRC) patients after failure of all standard treatments. In this single-center, real-world retrospective analysis of our platform for precision medicine, we mapped the molecular profiles of 60 mCRC patients. Tumor samples of the patients were analyzed using next-generation sequencing panels of mutation hotspots, microsatellite instability testing, and immunohistochemistry. All profiles were reviewed by a multidisciplinary team to provide a targeted treatment recommendation after consensus discussion. In total, we detected 166 mutations in 53 patients. The five most frequently found mutations were *TP53, KRAS, APC, PIK3CA,* and *PTEN*. In 28 cases (47% of all patients), a molecularly targeted therapy could be recommended. Eventually, 12 patients (20%) received the recommended therapy. Six patients (10%) had a clinical benefit. The median time to treatment failure was 3.1 months. Our study demonstrates the feasibility and applicability of using targeted therapies in daily clinical practice for heavily pretreated mCRC patients. This could be used as a targeted treatment option in half of the patients.

Keywords: molecular oncology; precision medicine; colorectal cancer; targeted therapy; molecular profiling

1. Introduction

Colorectal cancer (CRC) is one of the most frequent cancer types and is a major cause of mortality and morbidity. According to GLOBOCAN 2018, CRC is the fourth most common cancer disease throughout the world, equally affecting both men and women, with over 2 million new cases in 2018 [1]. It accounts for approximately 1 million deaths annually and 11% of all cancer deaths, ranking as the third most common cause of cancer death [1]. CRC particularly affects developed countries where inhabitants follow a western lifestyle that bears important risk factors for the carcinogenesis of CRC including alcohol intake, tobacco use, immoderate red and processed meat consumption, low intake of fiber, obesity, and a sedentary lifestyle [2].

In recent years, considerable effort has been made to explore the complex tumor biology of CRC and to expand and enrich the therapeutic armamentarium with new therapeutic agents. The therapeutic landscape for the management of metastatic CRC (mCRC) is rapidly evolving.

The development and application of monoclonal antibodies and tyrosine kinase inhibitors in addition to systemic cytotoxic (poly)chemotherapy have significantly improved the prognosis, median overall survival, and quality of life of mCRC patients [3,4].

Despite diagnostic and therapeutic advances in the management of mCRC, the 5-year survival rate for mCRC is approximately 14%, with a median overall survival of 30 months [5,6]. Moreover, after failure of standard therapy lines, therapeutic options are limited.

One way to offer treatment concepts for therapy refractory mCRC would be to analyze the molecular profile of tumors to identify actionable pathologic molecular alterations to develop an individually coordinated therapy plan. This individually tailored, tissue-agnostic molecular-based treatment approach is referred to as precision medicine in oncology or simply precision oncology [7,8].

In the last few years, more and more targeted therapy agents have been introduced for the management of several cancer diseases, such as trastuzumab in human epidermal growth factor receptor 2 (HER2 positive) breast cancer or gastric cancer [9,10], imatinib in in KIT+ gastrointestinal stromal tumor (GIST) [11], and B-rapidly accelerated fibrosarcoma (BRAF)-directed therapy with vemurafenib or dabrafenib/trametinib in melanoma [12].

Thus, exploring the molecular profile of mCRC may aid in the development of molecular targeted therapies and allow their efficacy to be tested.

In this study, we conducted a retrospective subgroup analysis of all 60 patients with advanced therapy refractory mCRC that had been enrolled and profiled via our special platform for precision medicine of the Comprehensive Cancer Centre of the Medical University of Vienna (CCC-MUV).

We sought to map the molecular profiles of mCRC to identify and target specific molecular alterations. We discuss the challenges, limitations, and the time to treatment failure (TTF) of precision medicine approaches in this patient group.

2. Methods

2.1. Patients and Design of the Precision Medicine Platform

All patients with heavily pretreated advanced metastatic CRC who had progressed to all standard treatment options and had undergone molecular profiling from June 2013 to June 2020 were included in this retrospective single-center study. This study was conducted at the Clinical Division of Oncology of the tertiary care university hospital Medical University of Vienna. Cancer patients refractory to all standard therapies were eligible for inclusion in our precision medicine platform, provided that tissue samples for molecular profiling were available. The specimens were either obtained by fresh tumor biopsy performed by physicians at the Department of Interventional Radiology or were provided by the archives of the Department of Pathology when tumor biopsy was not feasible. Patients had to have an Eastern Cooperative Oncology Group (ECOG) performance status of ≤1. All patients in this analysis had to be at least 18 years at the time of molecular analysis and had to provide informed consent before inclusion in our platform. Our precision medicine platform is not a clinical trial but intends to provide targeted therapy recommendations to patients where no standard antitumoral treatment is available. This analysis was approved by the Institutional Ethics Committee of the Medical University of Vienna (Nr. 1039/2017). The General Hospital of Vienna directly covered all costs for molecular profiling and targeted therapy provided the cancer patients had no further standard treatment options.

2.2. Evaluation of Outcome and Follow-Up

All patients with heavily pretreated advanced metastatic CRC who had progressed to all standard treatment options were confirmed by the response evaluation criteria in solid tumors 1.1 (RECIST 1.1) criteria [13]. These international criteria provide a basis for standardized and objective assessment of the change in tumor burden during treatment. The criteria distinguish four types of change:

- Complete response (CR): All target lesions disappear
- Partial response (PR): The sum of the longest diameter of target lesions decrease at least by 30%

- Stable disease (SD): Neither sufficient shrinkage to qualify for PR nor sufficient increase to qualify for PD
- Progressive disease (PD): The sum of the longest diameter of target lesions increase at least by 20%. PD means the tumor has become resistant to the therapy and, thus, the therapy has failed.

Follow-up was done every 8 to 12 weeks for outcome evaluation by radiological assessment depending on the respective therapy. If the patient did not appear on the follow-up date, we searched our electronic data processing system that is linked to the national death register to check and ascertain the death of the patient in the meantime.

2.3. Tissue Samples

Formalin-fixed, paraffin-embedded tissue samples from patients with metastatic CRC who had progressed through all standard therapy regimens were obtained from the archives of the Department of Pathology, Medical University of Vienna, Austria.

2.4. Cancer Gene Panel Sequencing

DNA was extracted from paraffin-embedded tissue blocks with a QIAamp Tissue KitTM (Qiagen, Hilden, Germany). From each tissue sample, 10 ng of DNA was provided for sequencing. The DNA library was created by multiplex polymerase chain reaction with the Ion AmpliSeq Cancer Hotspot Panel v2 (Thermo Fisher Scientific, Waltham, MA, USA), which covers mutation hotspots of 50 genes. The panel includes driver mutations, oncogenes, and tumor suppressor genes. In mid-2018, the gene panel was expanded using the 161-gene next-generation sequencing panel of Oncomine Comprehensive Assay v3 (Thermo Fisher Scientific, Waltham, MA, USA), which covers genetic alterations, gene amplifications, and gene fusions. The Ampliseq cancer hotspot panel was sequenced with an Ion PGM (Thermo Fisher) and the Oncomine Comprehensive Assay v3 on an Ion S5 sequencer (Thermo Fisher Scientific, Waltham, MA, USA). The generated sequencing data were analyzed afterwards with the help of Ion Reporter Software (Thermo Scientific Fisher). We referred to the BRCA Exchange, ClinVar, COSMIC, dbSNP, OMIM, and 1000 genomes for variant calling and classification. The variants were classified according to a five-tier system comprising pathogenic, likely pathogenic, uncertain significance, likely benign, or benign modifiers. This classification was based on the standards and guidelines for the interpretation of sequence variants of the American College of Medical Genetics and Genomics [14]. The pathogenic and likely pathogenic variants were taken into consideration for the recommendation of targeted therapy.

2.5. Immunohistochemistry

Immunohistochemistry (IHC) was performed using 2-μm-thin tissue sections that were read by a Ventana Benchmark Ultra stainer (Ventana Medical Systems, Tucson, AZ, USA). The following antibodies were applied: anaplastic lymphoma kinase (ALK) (clone 1A4; Zytomed, Berlin, Germany); CD20 (clone L26; Dako); CD30 (clone BerH2; Agilent Technologies, Vienna, Austria); DNA mismatch repair (MMR) proteins including MLH1 (clone M1, Ventana Medical Systems), PMS2 (clone EPR3947, Cell Marque, Rocklin, CA, USA), MSH2 (clone G219-1129, Cell Marque), and MSH6 (clone 44, Cell Marque); epidermal growth factor receptor (EGFR) (clone 3C6; Ventana); estrogen receptor (clone SP1; Ventana Medical Systems); human epidermal growth factor receptor 2 (HER2) (clone 4B5; Ventana Medical Systems); HER3 (clone SP71; Abcam, Cambridge, UK); C-kit receptor (KIT) (clone 9.7; Ventana Medical Systems); MET (clone SP44; Ventana); NTRK (clone EPR17341, Abcam); phosphorylated mammalian target of rapamycin (p-mTOR) (clone 49F9; Cell Signaling Technology, Danvers, MA, USA); platelet-derived growth factor alpha (PDGFRA) (rabbit polyclonal; Thermo Fisher Scientific); PDGFRB (clone 28E1, Cell Signaling Technology); programmed death-ligand 1 (PD-L1) (clone E1L3N; Cell Signaling Technology till mid-2018, as of mid-2018 the clone BSR90 from Nordic

Biosite, Stockholm, Sweden is used); progesterone receptor (clone 1E2; Ventana); phosphatase and tensin homolog (PTEN) (clone Y184; Abcam); and ROS1 (clone D4D6; Cell Signaling Technology).

To assess the immunostaining intensity for the antigens EGFR, p-mTOR, PDGFRA, PDGFRB, and PTEN, a combinative semiquantitative score for immunohistochemistry was used. The immunostaining intensity was graded from 0 to 3 (0 = negative, 1 = weak, 2 = moderate, and 3 = strong). To calculate the score, the intensity grade was multiplied by the percentage of corresponding positive cells: (maximum 300) = (% negative × 0) + (% weak × 1) + (% moderate × 2) + (% strong × 3).

The immunohistochemical staining intensity for HER2 was scored from 0 to 3+ (0 = negative, 1+ = negative, 2+ = positive, and 3+ = positive) pursuant to the scoring guidelines of the Dako HercepTestR from the company Agilent Technologies (Agilent Technologies, Vienna, Austria). In case of HER2 2+, a further test with HER2 in situ hybridization was performed to verify HER2 gene amplification.

Estrogen receptor and progesterone receptor staining were graded according to the Allred scoring system from 0 to 8. MET staining was scored from 0 to 3 (0 = negative, 1 = weak, 2 = moderate, and 3 = strong) based on a paper by Koeppen and coworkers. [15].

For PD-L1 protein expression, the tumor proportion score, which is the percentage of viable malignant cells showing membrane staining, was calculated. In addition, since 2019, the expression has also been determined by a combined positive score.

ALK, CD30, CD20, and ROS1 staining were classified as positive or negative based on the percentage of reactive tumor cells, however without graduation of the staining intensity. In ALK- or ROS1-positive cases, the presence of possible gene translocation was evaluated by fluorescence in situ hybridization (FISH).

All antibodies used in this study were validated and approved at the clinical institute of pathology of the Medical University of Vienna and are used in routine IHC staining for clinical purposes. The antibodies have been validated by proper positive and negative tissue controls and by non-IHC methods, such as immunoblotting and flow cytometry, to detect the respective epitopes of the antigens. For control, the use of the antibodies was optimized in terms of intensity, concentration, signal/noise ratio, incubation times, and blocking. The negative control involved omitting the primary antibody and substituting an isotype-specific antibody and serum at the exact same dilution and laboratory conditions as the primary antibody to preclude unspecific binding.

For positive control, the antibodies were shown not to cross-react with closely related molecules of the target epitope.

The status of microsatellite instability-high (MSI-H) was analyzed by the MSI Analysis System, version 1.1 (Promega Corporation, Madison, WI, USA).

2.6. Fluorescence in situ Hybridization (FISH)

FISH was only applied in selected cases to verify PTEN loss. FISH was performed with 4-μm-thick formalin-fixed, paraffin-embedded tissue sections. The following FISH probes were utilized: PTEN (10q23.31)/centromere 10 (ZytoVision, Bremerhaven, Germany). Two hundred cell nuclei were evaluated per tumor. The PTEN FISH was considered positive for PTEN gene loss with ≥30% of cells with only one or no PTEN signal. A chromosome 10 centromere FISH probe served as a control for the ploidy of chromosome 10.

2.7. Multidisciplinary Team for Precision Medicine

After thorough examination of the molecular profile of each tumor sample by a qualified molecular pathologist, the results were reviewed by a multidisciplinary team (MDT) that met every other week.

Members of the MDT included molecular pathologists, radiologists, clinical oncologists, surgical oncologists, and basic scientists. The MDT recommended targeted therapy based on the specific molecular profile of each patient, which included established pathological parameters. The targeted therapies included tyrosine kinase inhibitors, checkpoint inhibitors (e.g., anti-PD-L1 monoclonal antibodies), and growth factor receptor antibodies with or without endocrine therapy. The treatment recommendations by the MDT were prioritized using the level of evidence from high to low according to phase III to phase I trials.

In cases where more than one druggable molecular aberration was identified, the MDT recommended a therapy regimen to target as many molecular aberrations as possible, with special consideration given to the toxicity profile of each antitumoral agent and its potential interactions. Since all patients were given all available standard treatment options for their cancer disease prior to inclusion in our precision medicine platform, nearly all targeted agents suggested had off-label use. If the tumor profile and clinical characteristics of a patient met the requirements to be enrolled in a recruiting clinical trial for targeted therapies at our cancer center, patients were asked whether they wanted to participate in the respective trial, and trials adhered to ethical and regulatory guidelines.

2.8. Study Design and Statistics

The Fisher's exact test was employed to explore potential gender-specific differences regarding the therapy recommendation rate and the molecular profile. Student's *t*-test was applied to test differences in the outcome between tumor samples that were obtained during tumor biopsy versus specimens that were obtained during surgical resection. A *p*-value of less than 0.05 was considered to be statistically significant. For statistical analysis, the software package IBM SPSS Statistics Version 26 was used.

3. Results

3.1. Patient Characteristics

From the initiation of our platform for precision medicine in June 2013 until June 2020, we identified 60 patients with therapy refractory mCRC with no further standard treatment option available. These patients were all included in this subgroup analysis of our platform. All 60 patients were Caucasian, including 42 men (70%) and 18 women (30%). The cohort of mCRC patients comprised 47 patients (78%) with left-sided CRC and 13 patients (22%) with right-sided CRC (see Figure 1 for the patients' flow and Table 1 for the patient characteristics).

The median age at first diagnosis was 54.9 years (range: 16.9 to 81.2 years), and the median age at the time of molecular profiling was 57.9 years (range: 19.3 to 84.3 years). Tumor tissue used for molecular profiling was obtained by biopsy in 25 patients (42%) or during surgical treatment in the other 35 patients (58%). Biopsy was performed after failure of all standard treatment options. The median time interval between resection and molecular analysis of the tumor tissue was 11.9 months (range: 1–46 months). The median time interval between biopsy and completion of the molecular analysis of the tumor tissue was 31 days (range: 15–56 days). The median turnaround time between the initiation of molecular profiling and discussion by the MDT and molecular-based therapy initiation for the 12 patients who received the targeted therapy was 30 and 42 days, respectively. The median time interval between the initiation of molecular profiling and discussion of the MDT and molecular-based therapy initiation for the other patients ($n = 48$) was 29 days.

Twenty-one patients experienced a disease relapse. All of the patients had metastases, mainly in the liver, lungs, and bones. Seventeen patients had additional intraperitoneal dissemination of the CRC, causing peritoneal carcinomatosis. The patients received a median of three lines of prior palliative systemic chemotherapy, ranging from two to six lines. The palliative therapy regimens included FOLFOX + cetuximab, FOLFOX + bevacizumab, FOLFIRI + cetuximab, FOLFOX + panitumumab, FOLFIRI + panitumumab, FOLFOXIRI + bevacizumab, FOLFIRI + bevacizumab, FOLFIRI + aflibercept, FOLFIRI + ramucirumab, regorafenib, trifluridine/ tipiracil, and raltitrexed + oxaliplatin. Twenty-six patients (43%) had received at least four lines of palliative chemotherapy prior to molecular profiling.

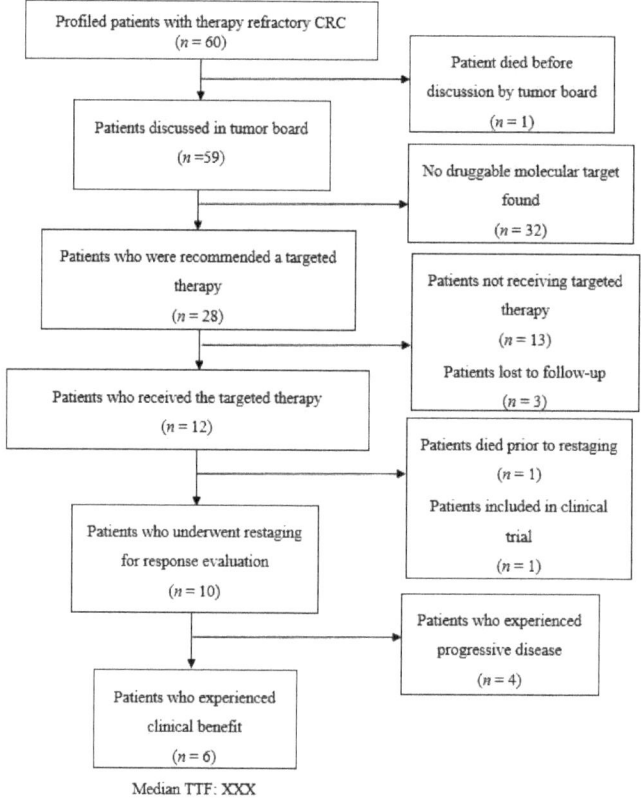

Figure 1. Flow chart of the 60 metastatic colorectal cancer (mCRC) patients.

3.2. Molecular Profile

In total, we detected 166 mutations in 53 patients (88%). The five most frequent mutations were *TP53* (*n* = 36; 60.0%), *KRAS* (*n* = 29; 48.3%), *APC* (*n* = 15; 25.0%), *PIK3CA* (*n* = 9; 15%), and *PTEN* (*n* = 8; 13.3%), which accounted for more than half of all mutations (58.4%). No mutations were detected in seven (12%) patients with our sequencing panel (Table 2). Seven gene fusions were identified in five patients: *FGFR3-TACC3* (*n* = 2), *FNDC3B-PIK3CA*, *SND1-BRAF*, *EIF3E-RSPO2*, *PTPRK-RSPO3*, and *WHSC1L1-FGFR1*. Moreover, we detected eight gene amplifications in six different tumor specimens, including *CCND2* (*n* = 3), *FLT3* (*n* = 3), *FGFR1*, and *MYC*.

Further, IHC revealed common expressions of phosphorylated mTOR and EGFR in 49 (82%) and 45 (75%) patients, respectively. The median IHC scores of mTOR and EGFR were 100 and 90, respectively. Ten patients (17%) had high levels of phosphorylated mTOR expression with an mTOR score between 200 and 300. EGFR expression was between 200 and 300 in nine patients (15%). In our cohort, two patients (3%) were HER2-positive and seven patients (12%) were HER3-positive. IHC identified six patients (10%) with a loss of PTEN, which was subsequently verified and characterized by FISH as heterozygous PTEN deletions. High expressions levels were also observed for MET (*n* = 28) and PDGFRA (*n* = 15). Four patients (7%) were given a status of MSI-H. In four patients, the PD-L1 combined positive score was ≥1. Three patients displayed a weak KIT expression. The expression of other markers was not observed. IHC and FISH could not be performed for one male patient due to insufficient tumor material. See Figure 2a–n.

Table 1. Patient characteristics ($n = 60$).

Patient Characteristics	Number
Median (range) age in years at first diagnosis	54.9 (16.9–81.2)
Median (range) age in years at time of molecular profiling	57.9 (19.3–84.3)
Male patients	42 (70%)
Female patients	18 (30%)
Caucasian	60 (100%)
Relapsed disease	23 (38%)
Metastatic disease	60 (100%)
Systemic chemotherapy received	60 (100%)
Prior chemotherapy regimens	2–6
Targeted therapy recommendations for patients	28 (47%)
• for male patients	19 (32%)
• for female patients	9 (15%)
Colorectal cancer localization	
• Right	13 (22%)
○ Cecum	6 (10%)
○ Ascending colon	5 (8%)
○ Transverse colon	2 (3%)
• Left	47 (78%)
○ Descending colon	2 (3%)
○ Sigmoid colon	27 (45%)
○ Rectum	18 (30%)
Number of metastasis	106
Liver metastasis	46 (43%)
Lung metastasis	32 (30%)
Peritoneal carcinomatosis	17 (16%)
Bone metastasis	4 (4%)
Cerebral metastasis	3 (3%)
Cutaneous metastasis	2 (3%)
Renal metastasis	1 (1%)
Splenic metastasis	1 (1%)
Number of mutations detected	166

3.3. Therapy Recommendations and Outcome

In 28 cases (47% of all patients), a molecularly targeted therapy was recommended. The other 32 patients (53%) did not qualify for targeted therapy due to the lack of actionable molecular targets. In over two-thirds of all recommendations ($n = 20/28$, 71.0%), the molecular-driven treatment approach was mainly derived from the molecular characteristics determined by immunohistochemistry. The 28 recommended targeted treatments included everolimus, pembrolizumab, nintedanib, cetuximab, vismodegib, vemurafenib, afatinib and trastuzumab combined with lapatinib, crizotinib, erlotinib, and sunitinib plus capecitabine. Table 3 describes the rationale for the recommended targeted therapy approaches. Eventually, 12 patients (20%) received the recommended targeted therapy. One patient with the KIT mutation was included in the clinical phase II trial SUNCAP and was treated with sunitinib and capecitabine. Another patient died prior to restaging. Finally, ten patients underwent radiological assessment (see Table 4). Four patients (7%) experienced progressive disease. Four patients with MSI-H status were given pembrolizumab and achieved a partial response ($n = 2$), complete response, and stable disease, respectively. Two patients treated with other targeted agents achieved a stable disease. Thus, the disease control rate was 10%. The three patients who achieved therapy response and one of the three patients who had stable disease experienced also an improvement in their quality of life due to an improvement in tumor pain intensity. The molecularly targeted therapies applied were pembrolizumab ($n = 4$), trastuzumab ($n = 2$), everolimus plus bevacizumab ($n = 2$), afatinib, everolimus, sunitinib plus capecitabine, and everolimus plus raltitrexed (see Tables 3 and 4 for further information). The median time to treatment failure (TTF) in patients who received the targeted therapy was 3.1 months (range: 0.3–30.6 months; see Figure 3 and Table 4). The median overall survival (mOS) of these 12 patients after initial diagnosis of mCRC was 50.1 months. The mOS after initiation of targeted therapy was 10.9 months (see Figure 4a,b). Three patients were lost to follow-up after the suggestion of molecular-driven targeted therapy. Thirteen patients (22%) did not receive the offered targeted therapy. Reasons for not applying the recommended targeted agent included the following: rapid deterioration of performance status ($n = 10$), death of patient ($n = 1$), the treating oncologist favoring another treatment regimen due to the clinical overall situation of the patients, or patients' refusal of any further treatment including targeted therapy options ($n = 2$).

Table 2. Genomic profile of the therapy refractory CRC patients ($n = 60$).

Mutated Genes	Number of Mutations	Percentage of Occurrence in Patients ($n = 60$)	Percentage of all Mutations (166 Mutations in Total)
TP53	36	60.0%	21.7%
KRAS	29	48.3%	17.5%
APC	15	25.0%	9.0%
PIK3CA	9	15.0%	5.4%
PTEN	8	13.3%	4.8%
ATM	5	8.3%	3.0%
SMAD4	5	8.3%	3.0%
NOTCH1	4	6.7%	2.4%
BRCA2	3	5.0%	1.8%
FBXW7	3	5.0%	1.8%
FGFR3	3	5.0%	1.8%
PTCH1	3	5.0%	1.8%
ERBB4	2	3.3%	1.2%
FANCA	2	3.3%	1.2%
GNAS	2	3.3%	1.2%
NOTCH3	2	3.3%	1.2%
POLE	2	3.3%	1.2%
SLX4	2	3.3%	1.2%
ALK	1	1.7%	0.6%
AR	1	1.7%	0.6%
ARID1A	1	1.7%	0.6%
ATRX	1	1.7%	0.6%
BRAF	1	1.7%	0.6%
CCND1	1	1.7%	0.6%
CDK12	1	1.7%	0.6%
CREBBP	1	1.7%	0.6%
CTNNB1	1	1.7%	0.6%
EGFR	1	1.7%	0.6%
ESR1	1	1.7%	0.6%
IDH1	1	1.7%	0.6%
JAK3	1	1.7%	0.6%
KDR	1	1.7%	0.6%
KIT	1	1.7%	0.6%
MAP2K1	1	1.7%	0.6%
MRE11A	1	1.7%	0.6%
MYC	1	1.7%	0.6%
NF1	1	1.7%	0.6%
NF2	1	1.7%	0.6%
NRAS	1	1.7%	0.6%
NTRK3	1	1.7%	0.6%
PALB2	1	1.7%	0.6%
RAD50	1	1.7%	0.6%
RB1	1	1.7%	0.6%
RICTOR	1	1.7%	0.6%
RNF43	1	1.7%	0.6%
SMARCA4	1	1.7%	0.6%
SMARCB1	1	1.7%	0.6%
SMO	1	1.7%	0.6%
TSC2	1	1.7%	0.6%

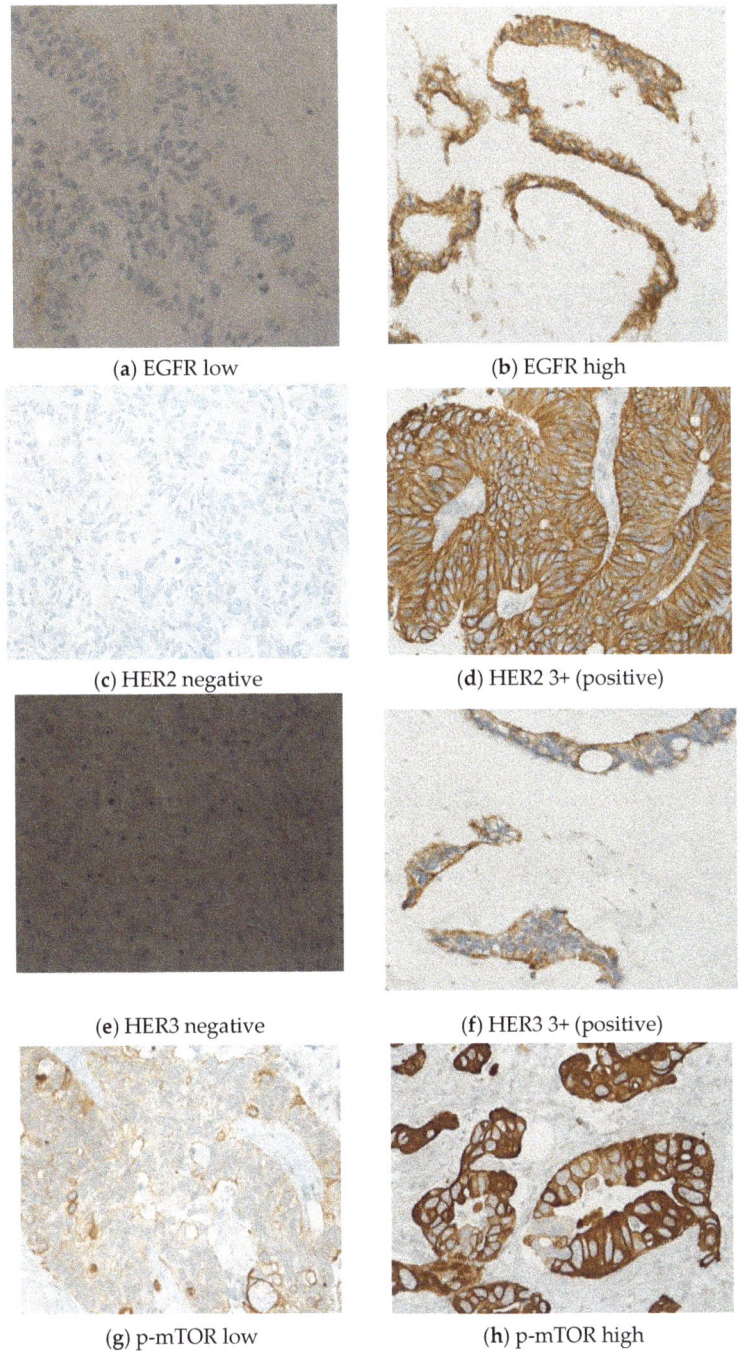

(a) EGFR low
(b) EGFR high
(c) HER2 negative
(d) HER2 3+ (positive)
(e) HER3 negative
(f) HER3 3+ (positive)
(g) p-mTOR low
(h) p-mTOR high

Figure 2. *Cont.*

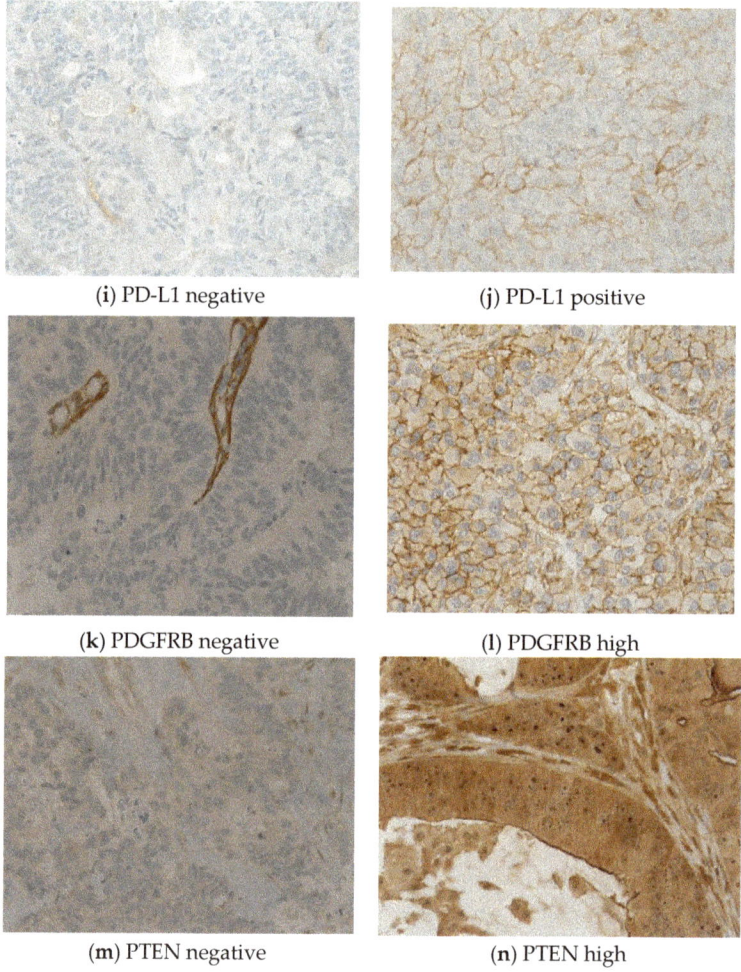

Figure 2. (**a–n**) These original images of immunohistochemistry show the differences between low and high expressions of various markers (Images by kind courtesy of Professor Dr. Müllauer).

Table 3. Rationale for targeted therapy recommendations.

Therapeutic Agent (Trading Name)	Targets	Overview of Current FDA Approval in Different Entities	Overview of Current EMA Approval in Different Entities	Number of Recommended and Received Cases and Responses
Pembrolizumab (Keytruda®)	PD-1, hypermutability	Melanoma, NSCLC, HNSCC, HL, Urothelial carcinoma, microsatellite instability-high cancer, gastric cancer, cervical cancer	Melanoma, NSCLC, HNSCC, HL, Urothelial carcinoma	-Recommended for and applied in 4 patients with MSI-H status: 1 patient achieved SD for 4.2 months; 2 patients achieved PR for 24.3 months and 30.5 months, respectively; 1 patient achieved CR for 27.5 months

Table 3. *Cont.*

Therapeutic Agent (Trading Name)	Targets	Overview of Current FDA Approval in Different Entities	Overview of Current EMA Approval in Different Entities	Number of Recommended and Received Cases and Responses
Cetuximab (Erbitux®)	EGFR	CRC, HNSCC	CRC, HNSCC	-Recommended in combination with everolimus for 1 patient with EGFR expression and *KRAS* wildtype (patient initially had a KRAS mutation) and loss of PTEN and mTOR expression -Recommended in combination with irinotecan for 1 patient with EGFR expression and the *KRAS* wildtype (patient had initially a KRAS mutation)
Vemurafenib (Zelboraf®)	BRAF V600E	BRAF V600E melanoma or NSCLC BRAF V600E melanoma	BRAF V600E melanoma or NSCLC BRAF V600E melanoma	-Recommended for 1 patient with BRAF V600E (recommended prior to the clinical phase III BEACON trial)
Nintedanib (Vargatef®, Ofev®)	FGFR, FLT3, PDGFR, VEGFR	Idiopathic pulmonary fibrosis	NSCLC	-Recommended for 3 patients: 1 patient had a FLT3 amplification, 1 patient had a FGFR3 fusion gene, and 1 patient had PDGFRA expression
Vismodegib (Erdivedge®)	SMO	Basal cell carcinoma	Basal cell carcinoma	-Recommended for 1 patient with the SMO mutation
Everolimus (Afinitor®)	mTOR expression	Breast cancer, PNET, RCC, renal angiomyolipoma, subependymal giant cell astrocytomas (SEGAs) with tuberous sclerosis complex (TSC)	Breast cancer, RCC, Neuroendocrine tumors of pancreatic, gastrointestinal, or lung origin	-Recommended for 6 patients with strong p-mTOR expression and PTEN deficiency: in one case, it was recommended and applied in combination with raltitrexed. The patient achieved SD for 9.0 months. In two cases, it was recommended and applied in combination with bevacizumab. Both patients experienced PD. In one case, it was recommended in combination with Cetuximab.
Trastuzumab (Herceptin®)	HER2	HER2+ breast cancer and gastric cancer	HER2+ breast cancer and gastric cancer	-Recommended for and applied in combination with lapatinib for 2 HER2+ patients: 1 patient achieved SD for 1.9 months and 1 patient experienced PD.
Lapatinib (Tykerb®, Tyverb®)	HER2, EGFR	HER2+ breast cancer	HER2+ breast cancer	-Recommended for and applied in combination with trastuzumab for 2 HER2+ patients: See trastuzumab.
Afatinib (Gilotrif®)	*EGFR*, HER1, HER2, HER3	NSCLC	NSCLC	-Recommended for 5 patients with HER3 expression and applied in 1 patient. The patient experienced PD.
Crizotinib (Xalkori®)	ALK, ROS1, HGFR, MET	ROS1+ or ALK+ NSCLC	ROS1+ or ALK+ NSCLC	Recommended for 2 patients with MET expression
Erlotinib (Tarceva®)	EGFR	NSCLC, PDAC	NSCLC, PDAC	-Recommended for 1 patient with the EGFR mutation
Sunitinib (Sutent®)	PDGFR, KIT, VEGFR, RET, FLT3	RCC, PDAC, GIST	RCC, PDAC, GIST	-Recommended in combination with capecitabine for 1 patient with the KIT mutation: the patient was enrolled in the phase II SUNCAP trial.

ABL1, Abelson murine leukemia viral oncogene homolog 1; AML, acute myeloid leukemia; ALL, acute lymphatic leukemia; BCR, breakpoint cluster region; CML, chronic myeloid leukemia; CRC, colorectal cancer; EGFR epidermal growth factor receptor; EMA, European Medicines Agency; FDA, Food and Drug Administration; FLT3, fms like tyrosine kinase 3; GIST, gastrointestinal stromal tumor; GNRHR, gonadotropin-releasing hormone receptor; HER2, human epidermal growth factor receptor 2; HL, Hodgkin lymphoma; HNSCC, head and neck squamous cell carcinoma; MCL, mantle cell lymphoma; MDS, myelodysplastic syndrome; MPD, myeloproliferative disorder; NSCLC, non-small-cell lung carcinoma; PD, progressive disease; PD-1, programmed cell death protein 1; PDAC, pancreatic ductal adenocarcinoma; PDGFR, platelet-derived growth factor receptor; Ph+: Philadelphia chromosome positive; p-mTOR, phosphorylated mammalian target of rapamycin; RCC, renal cell carcinoma; RET, rearranged during transfection; SD, stable disease; VEGFR, vascular endothelial growth factor.

Table 4. Characteristics of the CRC patients receiving the molecular-based targeted therapy recommendation ($n = 12$).

Number, Gender, Localization of CRC	Detected Mutations; Gene Fusions	Immunohistochemistry	Applied Targeted Therapy	Age (in Years) at Time of Molecular Profiling	TTF in Months	Therapy Response	Cause of Therapy Termination
1 Male Sigmoid carcinoma	KRAS	EGFR score = 90, MET score = 3, p-mTOR score = 110, loss of PTEN	Everolimus combined with bevacizumab	65.5	2.8	PD	PD
2 Male Sigmoid carcinoma	NRAS, PTEN	p-mTOR score = 65, loss of PTEN	Everolimus combined with raltitrexed	49.0	9.1	SD	PD
3 Male Sigmoid carcinoma	No mutations detected	MSI-H	Pembrolizumab	53.2	24.3	PR	PD
4 Male Carcinoma of the ascending colon	APC, PTEN, TP53	MSI-H, EGFR score = 180, MET score = 3, p-mTOR score = 80	Pembrolizumab	48.7	30.6	PR	PD
5 Male Cecum carcinoma	APC, KRAS, TP53	EGFR score = 30, HER3 score = 3, MET score = 2, p-mTOR = 100, EGFR score = 280	Afatinib	55.6	2.3	PD	PD
6 Male Rectal cancer	PIK3CA, TP53	HER2 score = 2, HER3 score = 3, MET score = 2, p-mTOR = 240	Trastuzumab combined with lapatinib	56.2	1.9	SD	PD
7 Male Sigmoid carcinoma	AR, ARID1A, ATM, PALB2, PIK3CA, RNF43; FGFR3–TACC3	MSI-H EGFR score = 200, PTEN score = 100, p-mTOR = 240	Pembrolizumab	58.3	4.2	SD	PD
8 Female Sigmoid carcinoma	CTNNB1, KRAS, PTEN, RB1, TP53	MSI-H,	Pembrolizumab	42.0	27.5	CR	Relapse
9 Female Sigmoid carcinoma	No mutations detected	HER2 score = 3, p-mTOR = 120	Trastuzumab combined with lapatinib	50.3	3.1	PD	PD
10 Female Rectal cancer	BRCA2, KRAS, POLE, PTCH1, RAD50, TP53	EGFR score = 50, p-mTOR = 60,	Everolimus combined with bevacizumab	57.0	1.7	PD	PD

Table 4. *Cont.*

Number, Gender, Localization of CRC	Detected Mutations; Gene Fusions	Immunohistochemistry	Applied Targeted Therapy	Age (in Years) at Time of Molecular Profiling	TTF in Months	Therapy Response	Cause of Therapy Termination
11 Female Sigmoid carcinoma	TP53	EGFR score = 110, HER3 score = 2, MET score = 1, p-mTOR = 240, loss of PTEN	Everolimus	19.3	0.3	n.a.	Death
12 Male Carcinoma of the ascending colon	KIT, KRAS, TP53	EGFR score = 50, MET score = 2, p-mTOR = 40,	Sunitinib combined with capecitabine; The patient was enrolled in the phase II SUNCAP trial.	70.0	n.a.	n.a.	n.a.

n.a., not applicable; AR, androgen receptor; CPS, combined prognostic score; ECOG PS, Eastern Cooperative Oncology Group performance status; EGFR epidermal growth factor receptor; MSI-H, microsatellite instability-high; PD, progressive disease; PDL1, programmed death ligand 1; PDGFRA, platelet-derived growth factor receptor alpha; p-mTOR, phosphorylated mammalian target of rapamycin; SD, stable disease, PTEN, phosphatase and tensin homolog; TPS, tumor positive score.

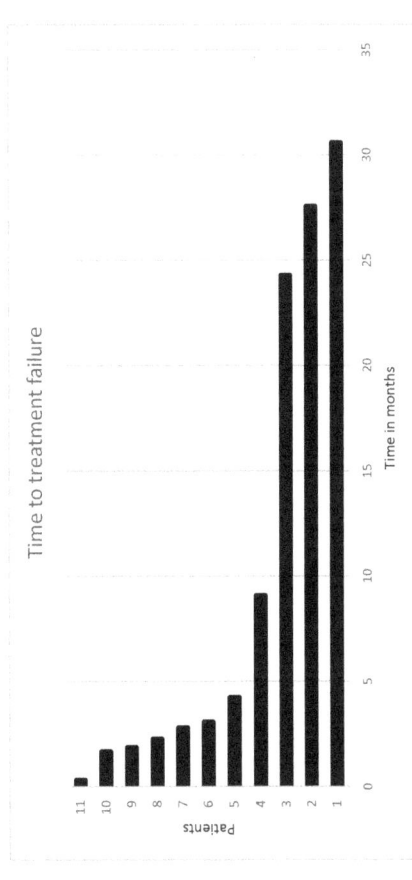

Figure 3. Time to treatment failure (TTF) in 11 CRC patients who received the recommended targeted therapy: the median time to treatment failure was 3.1 months.

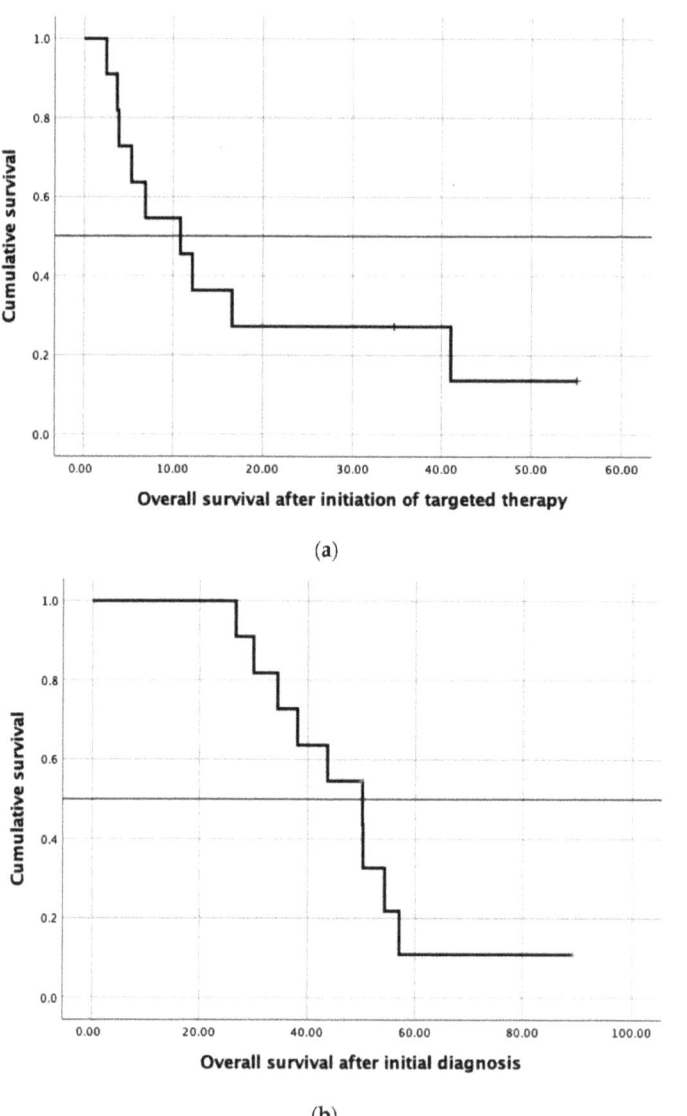

Figure 4. (a) Kaplan–Meier survival curve showing overall survival after initiation of targeted therapy in twelve patients receiving the targeted therapy and (b) Kaplan–Meier survival curve showing overall survival after initial diagnosis of mCRC in twelve patients receiving the targeted therapy.

Three tumor specimens from the ten patients who underwent radiological assessment were obtained during a conventional tumor biopsy. Two of these three patients experienced progressive disease, and one patient achieved stable disease. The tumor sample of the remaining seven patients was yielded during surgical resection of the primary tumor. We found no significant difference between tumor samples obtained during tumor biopsy versus surgical resection in terms of TTF ($p = 0.319$) and mOS ($p = 0.396$).

According to the Fisher's exact test, the gender-specific differences regarding the 28 targeted therapy recommendations were not statistically significant ($p = 0.516$).

4. Discussions

In our study, we recommended 28 molecularly targeted therapies based on the respective individual molecular profile of heavily pretreated mCRC patients. Thus, precision medicine approaches were found to be feasible and implementable in daily clinical routine in approximately half of the patients who had no further standard treatment option. In over two-thirds of all recommendations, the molecular-based targeted treatment approach was mainly derived from the molecular characteristics determined by immunohistochemistry. This fact underlines the major clinical relevance of immunohistochemistry in precision medicine as immunohistochemistry and next-generation sequencing complement each other. This could be very useful as sequencing panels are updated and enlarged routinely, adding valuable information for treatment decision making.

However, one important limitation of this study was that other parts of the molecular portrait were not analyzed. The molecular profile of a tumor is intricate and complex and goes beyond these two techniques. Comprehensive mapping of the molecular profile is multilayered and multi-faceted and includes many other aspects, including genomics, epigenomics, transcriptomics, proteomics including phospho- and glycoproteomics, metabolomics, epigenetics, and microbiomics [16]. The processing and integration of these extremely large quantities of data and their translation into targeted therapy recommendations is a grand challenge that scientists and clinicians are confronted with. There are close links among all involved disciplines to achieve common objectives. Further, CRC is characterized by highly dynamic and complex molecular intratumoral and intertumoral heterogeneity that changes both temporally and spatially [16–21]. The tumor tissue used for molecular profiling was obtained by biopsy in 25 patients (42%) or during surgical treatment in the other 35 patients (58%). Biopsy was performed after failure of all standard treatment options. Whenever possible, we used metastatic tissue for molecular profiling, which was particularly suited when fresh biopsies were obtained. If this approach was not feasible, e.g., if the anatomic site was not suitable for biopsy, we used the information obtained from the primary tumor site. Despite potential spatial heterogeneity, we assumed that most of the genetic aberrations in the primary cancer were also present at the metastatic site. Studies have shown that there is a high biomarker concordance between primary colorectal cancer and its metastases [22]. We found no significant difference between tumor samples obtained during tumor biopsy versus surgical resection in terms of TTF. However, the number of patients (n = 10) who underwent radiological response assessment after application of the targeted therapy was too limited to examine the influence of biomarker concordance on the outcome. Thus, further clinical trials and studies are required to examine the degree of biomarker concordance between primary cancer and metastases.

In our cohort, the five most frequent mutations, *TP53*, *KRAS*, *APC*, *PIK3CA*, and *PTEN*, together accounted for more than 50% percent of all detected mutations. Except for PIK3CA mutations, there are still no molecularly targeted therapies that directly target the mutations in *TP53*, *KRAS*, *APC*, and *PTEN*. Thus, there is an unmet clinical need for the inhibition of these genetic aberrations. The rest of the detected mutations were of low frequency (below 10%) and reflect the well-known molecular heterogeneity and diversity of CRC. The detected genetic aberrations are in line with the results of previous studies [23–25].

Moreover, a growing body of evidence shows that the antitumoral therapy itself may affect, influence, and drive tumor molecular evolution [26–28]. A prime example of this phenomenon is the recommendation of cetuximab for two patients who were initially KRAS-mutated and were therefore not treated with an anti-EGFR therapy; however, at the time of molecular profiling, they had developed the RAS wildtype [29].

One way to monitor the dynamic molecular landscape of cancer disease would be the utilization of real-time liquid biopsy to adapt antitumoral therapy according to the current molecular portrait [30].

To this end, the multicenter clinical phase II trial MoliMor (EudraCT number: 2019–003714–14) is evaluating the efficacy and safety of intermittent addition of cetuximab to a FOLFIRI-based first-line therapy to patients with RAS-mutant mCRC at diagnosis who convert to the RAS wildtype using monitoring of the RAS mutation status by liquid biopsy. Liquid biopsy may be also suitable for therapy response and for the detection of early signs of therapy resistance. Furthermore, the application of liquid biopsy may also help to reduce the long turnaround time of one month from biopsy of the tumor tissue to completion of the molecular profile. One of the main limitations of this study was the relatively long turnaround time between biopsy and completion of molecular analysis and between initiation of molecular profiling and discussion of the MDT and molecular-based therapy initiations with 30 and 42 days, respectively.

Time is a highly critical factor in the therapeutic management of mCRC, and a turnaround time of over one month without administration of effective therapy means that the mCRC progresses further. The growing metastases, particularly liver metastases, may lead to liver failure, increasing bilirubin values, and rapid health deterioration, making administration of the recommended targeted therapy impossible. From 28 molecularly targeted therapy recommendations, less than half of the patients eventually received the therapy. The TTF of 3.1 months and the disease control rate of 10% are modest outcomes. One reason for these modest outcomes may be that, due to the long turnaround time, there was not enough time for the targeted therapy to display its full potential. Other reasons may be the aforementioned tumor heterogeneity and the non-consideration of other aspects of the molecular profile as an important limitation. Interestingly, the three patients who achieved therapy response and one of the three patients who had stable disease experienced also improvements in their quality of life due to improvements in tumor pain intensity.

Furthermore, the design of this study is retrospective and it may be associated—in contrast to a prospective randomized controlled trial—with several limitations, including selection bias, insufficient documentation of clinical data, inadequate consideration of potential confounders, and the lack of randomization.

An additional limiting factor is that this retrospective study was conducted at a single center with a relatively small number of patients. It is difficult to demonstrate treatment efficacy, treatment difference, or certain findings in a small sample. In addition, single-center studies lack external validity to support or confirm the findings. Further research and clinical trials are warranted to evaluate the role and value of precision medicine for the management of mCRC patients.

In our study, we paid close attention to potential gender-specific differences. We did not find any gender-specific differences regarding the 28 targeted therapy recommendations.

Our study emphasizes the relevance and efficacy of pembrolizumab, even in metastatic patients with heavily pretreated therapy refractory mCRC who were classified as MSI-H.

It was shown that MSI-H status is a favorable prognostic factor at early local stages, particularly in stage II [31]. However, in stage IV CRC, MSI-H confers an inferior prognosis when compared to microsatellite stable metastatic CRC [32–34].

In our limited subset of patients with MSI-H, we administered pembrolizumab to four patients as no other druggable target could be derived from the molecular profile. Although MSI-H is not a favorable predictive marker in stage IV CRC, we achieved an impressive response with one complete remission, two partial remissions, and one stabile disease.

Pembrolizumab was the first tissue-agnostic treatment that was granted approval by the Food and Drug Administration (FDA) by mid-2017 for patients with unresectable or metastatic MSI-H or with mismatch repair deficient (dMMR) solid tumors that progress following prior treatment and who have no satisfactory alternative treatment options or those with MSI-H or dMMR colorectal cancer that progresses following treatment with a fluoropyrimidine, oxaliplatin, and irinotecan [35]. However, its use for MSI-H patients has not been still approved by the European Medicines Agency (EMA), and it was applied in off-label form in this study.

Taken together, the management of mCRC patients poses several major challenges, including the long turnaround time and the complex molecular heterogeneity of CRC. Our study underscores the relevance of immunohistochemistry and underlines the importance of time as a highly critical factor in precision medicine. Based on our study, molecular-based treatment approaches can be of clinical benefit in select heavily pretreated mCRC patients. In this study, the overall benefit for precision medicine approaches was limited and the TTF was relatively modest. However, precision medicine is a rapidly evolving field. In the next few years, technical advances will allow us to employ larger gene panels to cover and identify more mutations, amplifications, deletions, and gene fusions in a shorter period of time. The development of new and potent molecularly targeted therapies together with technical progresses in molecular profiling allow us to hope that, in the future, we may be able to yield deep and durable responses in heavily pretreated mCRC patients.

Author Contributions: Conceptualization, H.T., R.M.M. and G.W.P.; methodology, H.T., R.M.M., and G.W.P.; formal analysis, H.T., R.M.M., L.M., F.E., A.K.-W. and G.W.P.; investigation, H.T., R.M.M., G.W.P.; resources, H.T., R.M.M., L.M., F.E., A.K.-W. and G.W.P.; data curation, H.T., R.M.M., L.M., F.E. and G.W.P.; writing—original draft preparation, H.T.; writing—review and editing, all authors.; visualization, H.T.; supervision, R.M.M. and G.W.P.; project administration, H.T., R.M.M., L.M. and G.W.P. All authors have read and agreed to the published version of the manuscript.

Funding: This research received no external funding.

Conflicts of Interest: The authors declare no conflict of interest.

References

1. Bray, F.; Ferlay, J.; Soerjomataram, I.; Siegel, R.L.; Torre, L.A.; Jemal, A. Global cancer statistics 2018, GLOBOCAN estimates of incidence and mortality worldwide for 36 cancers in 185 countries. *CA Cancer J. Clin.* **2018**, *68*, 394–424. [CrossRef]
2. Durko, L.; Małecka-Panas, E. Lifestyle Modifications and Colorectal Cancer. *Curr. Colorectal. Cancer Rep.* **2014**, *10*, 45–54. [CrossRef]
3. Modest, D.P.; Pant, S.; Sartore-Bianchi, A. Treatment sequencing in metastatic colorectal cancer. *Eur. J. Cancer* **2019**, *109*, 70–83. [CrossRef]
4. Tran, N.H.; Cavalcante, L.L.; Lubner, S.J.; Mulkerin, D.L.; LoConte, N.K.; Clipson, L.; Matkowskyj, K.A.; Deming, D.A. Precision medicine in colorectal cancer: The molecular profile alters treatment strategies. *Ther. Adv. Med. Oncol.* **2015**, *7*, 252–262. [CrossRef] [PubMed]
5. Lamarre, J.; Cervantes, A.; Adam, R.; Sobrero, A.; Van Krieken, J.H.; Aderka, D.; Aguilar, E.A.; Bardelli, A.; Benson, A.; Bodoky, G.; et al. ESMO consensus guidelines for the management of patients with metastatic colorectal cancer. *Ann. Oncol.* **2016**, *27*, 1386–1422.
6. Wang, J.; Li, S.; Liu, Y.; Zhang, C.; Li, H.; Lai, B. Metastatic patterns and survival outcomes in patients with stage IV colon cancer: A population-based analysis. *Cancer Med.* **2020**, *9*, 361–373. [CrossRef] [PubMed]
7. Garraway, L.A.; Verweij, J.; Ballman, K.V. Precision oncology: An overview. *J. Clin. Oncol.* **2013**, *31*, 1803–1805. [CrossRef] [PubMed]
8. Schwartzberg, L.; Kim, E.S.; Liu, D.; Schrag, D. Precision Oncology: Who, How, What, When, and When Not? *Am. Soc. Clin. Oncol. Educ. Book* **2017**, *37*, 160–169. [CrossRef]
9. Bang, Y.-J.; Van Cutsem, E.; Feyereislova, A.; Chung, H.C.; Shen, L.; Sawaki, A.; Lordick, F.; Ohtsu, A.; Omuro, Y.; Satoh, T.; et al. Trastuzumab in combination with chemotherapy versus chemotherapy alone for treatment of HER2-positive advanced gastric or gastro-oesophageal junction cancer (ToGA): A phase 3, open-label, randomised controlled trial. *Lancet* **2010**, *376*, 687–697. [CrossRef]
10. Slamon, D.J.; Eiermann, W.; Robert, N.; Pienkowski, T.; Martin, M.; Press, M.; Mackey, J.; Glaspy, J.; Chan, A.; Pawlicki, M.; et al. Adjuvant trastuzumab in HER2-positive breast cancer. *N. Engl. J. Med.* **2011**, *365*, 1273–1283. [CrossRef]
11. Blanke, C.D.; Rankin, C.; Demetri, G.D.; Ryan, C.W.; Von Mehren, M.; Benjamin, R.S.; Raymond, A.K.; Bramwell, V.H.; Baker, L.H.; Maki, R.G.; et al. Phase III randomized, intergroup trial assessing imatinib mesylate at two dose levels in patients with unresectable or metastatic gastrointestinal stromal tumors expressing the kit receptor tyrosine kinase: S0033. *J. Clin. Oncol.* **2008**, *26*, 626–632. [CrossRef] [PubMed]

12. Hauschild, A.; Grob, J.-J.; Demidov, L.V.; Jouary, T.; Gutzmer, R.; Millward, M.; Rutkowski, P.; Blank, C.U.; Miller, W.H.; Kaempgen, E.; et al. Dabrafenib in BRAF-mutated metastatic melanoma: A multicentre, open-label, phase 3 randomised controlled trial. *Lancet* **2012**, *380*, 358–365. [CrossRef]
13. Eisenhauer, E.A.; Therasse, P.; Bogaerts, J.; Schwartz, L.H.; Sargent, D.; Ford, R.; Dancey, J.; Arbuck, S.; Gwyther, S.; Mooney, M.; et al. New response evaluation criteria in solid tumours: Revised RECIST guideline (version 1.1). *Eur. J. Cancer* **2009**, *45*, 228–247. [CrossRef] [PubMed]
14. Richards, S.; Aziz, N.; Bale, S.; Bick, D.; Das, S.; Gastier-Foster, J.; Grody, W.W.; Hegde, M.; Lyon, E.; Spector, E.; et al. Standards and guidelines for the interpretation of sequence variants: A joint consensus recommendation of the American College of Medical Genetics and Genomics and the Association for Molecular Pathology. *Genet. Med.* **2015**, *17*, 405–424. [CrossRef]
15. Koeppen, H.; Yu, W.; Zha, J.; Pandita, A.; Pandita, A.; Rangell, L.; Raja, R.; Mohan, S.; Patel, R.; Patel, R.; et al. Biomarker analyses from a placebo-controlled phase II study evaluating erlotinib+/−onartuzumab in advanced non-small cell lung cancer: MET expression levels are predictive of patient benefit. *Clin. Cancer Res.* **2014**, *20*, 4488–4498. [CrossRef]
16. Merlano, M.C.; Granetto, C.; Fea, E.; Ricci, V.; Garrone, O. Heterogeneity of colon cancer: From bench to bedside. *ESMO Open* **2017**, *2*, e000218. [CrossRef]
17. Molinari, C.; Marisi, G.; Passardi, A.; Matteucci, L.; De Maio, G.; Ulivi, P. Heterogeneity in Colorectal Cancer: A Challenge for Personalized Medicine? *Int. J. Mol. Sci.* **2018**, *19*, 3733. [CrossRef]
18. Punt, C.J.A.; Koopman, M.; Vermeulen, L. From tumour heterogeneity to advances in precision treatment of colorectal cancer. *Nat. Rev. Clin. Oncol.* **2017**, *14*, 235–246. [CrossRef]
19. Árnadóttir, S.S.; Jeppesen, M.; Lamy, P.; Bramsen, J.B.; Nordentoft, I.; Knudsen, M.; Vang, S.; Madsen, M.R.; Thastrup, O.; Thastrup, J.; et al. Characterization of genetic intratumor heterogeneity in colorectal cancer and matching patient-derived spheroid cultures. *Mol. Oncol.* **2018**, *12*, 132–147. [CrossRef]
20. Jones, H.G.; Jenkins, G.; Williams, N.; Griffiths, P.; Chambers, P.; Beynon, J.; Harris, D. Genetic and Epigenetic Intra-tumour Heterogeneity in Colorectal Cancer. *World J. Surg.* **2017**, *41*, 1375–1383. [CrossRef]
21. Del Carmen, S.; Sayagués, J.M.; Bengoechea, O.; Anduaga, M.F.; Alcazar, J.A.; Gervas, R.; García, J.; Orfao, A.; Bellvis, L.M.; Sarasquete, M.-E.; et al. Spatio-temporal tumor heterogeneity in metastatic CRC tumors: A mutational-based approach. *Oncotarget* **2018**, *9*, 34279–34288. [CrossRef] [PubMed]
22. Bhullar, D.; Barriuso, J.; Mullamitha, S.; Saunders, M.; O'Dwyer, S.; Aziz, O. Biomarker concordance between primary colorectal cancer and its metastases. *EBioMedicine* **2019**, *40*, 363–374. [CrossRef] [PubMed]
23. Armaghany, T.; Wilson, J.D.; Chu, Q.; Mills, G. Genetic alterations in colorectal cancer. *Gastrointest Cancer Res.* **2012**, *5*, 19–27. [PubMed]
24. Munteanu, I.; Mastalier, B. Genetics of colorectal cancer. *J. Med. Life* **2014**, *7*, 507–511.
25. Sameer, A.S. Colorectal cancer: Molecular mutations and polymorphisms. *Front. Oncol.* **2013**, *3*, 114. [CrossRef]
26. Venkatesan, S.; Swanton, C.; Taylor, B.S.; Costello, J.F. Treatment-Induced Mutagenesis and Selective Pressures Sculpt Cancer Evolution. *Cold Spring Harb Perspect Med.* **2017**, *7*, a026617. [CrossRef]
27. Ibragimova, M.K.; Tsyganov, M.M.; Litviakov, N.V. Natural and Chemotherapy-Induced Clonal Evolution of Tumors. *Biochemistry* **2017**, *82*, 413–425. [CrossRef]
28. Testa, U.; Pelosi, E.; Castelli, G. Colorectal cancer: Genetic abnormalities, tumor progression, tumor heterogeneity, clonal evolution and tumor-initiating cells. *Med. Sci.* **2018**, *6*, 31. [CrossRef]
29. Benjamin, L.E. KRAS mutation status is predictive of response to cetuximab therapy in colorectal cancer. *Cancer Res.* **2006**, *66*, 3992–3995. [CrossRef]
30. Vitiello, P.P.; De Falco, V.; Giunta, E.F.; Ciardiello, F.; Cardone, C.; Vitale, P.; Zanaletti, N.; Borrelli, C.; Poliero, L.; Terminiello, M.; et al. Clinical Practice Use of Liquid Biopsy to Identify RAS/BRAF Mutations in Patients with Metastatic Colorectal Cancer (mCRC): A Single Institution Experience. *Cancers* **2019**, *11*, 1504. [CrossRef]
31. Saridaki, Z.; Souglakos, J.; Georgoulias, V. Prognostic and predictive significance of MSI in stages II/III colon cancer. *World J. Gastroenterol.* **2014**, *20*, 6809–6814. [CrossRef] [PubMed]
32. Venderbosch, S.; Nagtegaal, I.D.; Maughan, T.S.; Smith, C.G.; Cheadle, J.P.; Fisher, D.; Kaplan, R.; Quirke, P.; Seymour, M.T.; Richman, S.D.; et al. Mismatch repair status and BRAF mutation status in metastatic colorectal cancer patients: A pooled analysis of the CAIRO, CAIRO2, COIN, and FOCUS studies. *Clin. Cancer Res.* **2014**, *20*, 5322–5330. [CrossRef] [PubMed]

33. Aasebø, K.; Dragomir, A.; Sundström, M.; Mezheyeuski, A.; Edqvist, P.; Eide, G.E.; Ponten, F.; Pfeiffer, P.; Glimelius, B.; Sorbye, H. Consequences of a high incidence of microsatellite instability and BRAF-mutated tumors: A population-based cohort of metastatic colorectal cancer patients. *Cancer Med.* **2019**, *8*, 3623–3635. [CrossRef] [PubMed]
34. Shulman, K.; Barnett-Griness, O.; Friedman, V.; Greenson, J.K.; Gruber, S.B.; Lejbkowicz, F.; Rennert, G. Outcomes of Chemotherapy for Microsatellite Instable–High Metastatic Colorectal Cancers. *JCO Precis. Oncol.* **2018**, *2*, 1–10. [CrossRef]
35. Marcus, L.; Lemery, S.J.; Keegan, P.; Pazdur, R. FDA Approval Summary: Pembrolizumab for the Treatment of Microsatellite Instability-High Solid Tumors. *Clin. Cancer Res.* **2019**, *25*, 3753–3758. [CrossRef] [PubMed]

Publisher's Note: MDPI stays neutral with regard to jurisdictional claims in published maps and institutional affiliations.

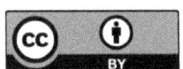

© 2020 by the authors. Licensee MDPI, Basel, Switzerland. This article is an open access article distributed under the terms and conditions of the Creative Commons Attribution (CC BY) license (http://creativecommons.org/licenses/by/4.0/).

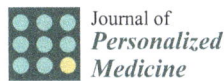

Article

Prognostic Impact of the Neutrophil-to-Lymphocyte and Lymphocyte-to-Monocyte Ratio, in Patients with Rectal Cancer: A Retrospective Study of 1052 Patients

Zsolt Zoltán Fülöp [1,†], Réka Linda Fülöp [1,†], Simona Gurzu [2,3,*], Tivadar Bara, Jr. [1], József Tímár [4], Emőke Drágus [5] and Ioan Jung [2]

[1] Department of Surgery, George Emil Palade University of Medicine, Pharmacy, Sciences and Technology, 540139 Targu Mures, Romania; zsolt_fulop15@yahoo.com (Z.Z.F.); rekafulop@ymail.com (R.L.F.); btibi_ms@yahoo.com (T.B.J.)
[2] Department of Pathology, George Emil Palade University of Medicine, Pharmacy, Sciences and Technology, 38 Gheorghe Marinescu Street, 540139 Targu Mures, Romania; jungjanos@studium.ro
[3] Research Center (CCAMF), George Emil Palade University of Medicine, Pharmacy, Sciences and Technology, 540139 Targu Mures, Romania
[4] Second Department of Pathology, National Institute of Oncology, Faculty of Medicine, Semmelweis University, H-1085 Budapest, Hungary; jtimar@gmail.com
[5] Department of Urology, Clinical County Hospital, 540167 Targu Mures, Romania; d.emoke_29@yahoo.com
* Correspondence: simonagurzu@yahoo.com; Tel.: +40-745-673550; Fax: +40-265-210407
† These two authors equally contributed to the paper.

Received: 27 August 2020; Accepted: 14 October 2020; Published: 16 October 2020

Abstract: Despite the description of several new prognostic markers, colorectal cancer still represents the third most frequent cause of cancer-related death. As immunotherapy is considered a therapeutic alternative in such patients, neutrophil-to-lymphocyte (NLR) and lymphocyte-to-monocyte ratio (LMR) are hypothesized to provide reliable prognostic information. A retrospective study was conducted on 1052 patients operated on during 2013–2019 in two clinical hospitals from Hungary and Romania. Inclusion criteria targeted patients over 18 years old, diagnosed with rectal cancer, with preoperatively defined NLR and LMR. The overall survival rate, along with clinical and histopathological data, was evaluated. Overall survival was significantly associated with increased NLR ($p = 0.03$) and decreased LMR ($p = 0.04$), with cut-off values of 3.11 and 3.39, respectively. The two parameters were inversely correlated ($p < 0.0001$). There was no statistically significant association between tumor stage and NLR or LMR ($p = 0.30$, $p = 0.06$, respectively). The total mesorectal excision was especially obtained in cases with low NLR ($p = 0.0005$) and high LMR ($p = 0.0009$) values. A significant association was also seen between preoperative chemoradiotherapy and high NLR ($p = 0.0001$) and low LMR ($p = 0.0001$). In patients with rectal cancer, the preoperative values of NLR and LMR can be used as independent prognostic parameters. An NLR value of ≥3.11 can be used to indicate the response to preoperative chemoradiotherapy, but a low chance of sphincter preservation or obtaining a complete TME. Higher values of NLR and lower values of LMR require a more attentive preoperative evaluation of the mesorectum.

Keywords: neutrophil-to-lymphocyte ratio; lymphocyte-to-monocyte ratio; prognosis; rectal cancer; mesorectum; sphincter preserving

1. Introduction

Colorectal cancer (CRC) is responsible for about 10% of all diagnosed malignant tumors and cancer-related deaths worldwide [1]. Regarding its diagnosis between genders, it is the third most common cancer in men and the second most frequent in women [1]. Approximately one-third of CRC cases are diagnosed within the rectum [2].

In 1863, Rudolf Virchow first described a possible association between malignant tumors and inflammation, highlighting the role of the density of white blood cells in carcinoma behavior [3–6]. Recently, multiple studies have investigated the role of the systemic inflammatory response (SIR) in carcinogenesis, progression, and prognosis of different cancer types [6–8], but the results are controversial. The SIR is defined by several parameters, including the neutrophil-to-lymphocyte ratio (NLR) and lymphocyte-to-monocyte ratio (LMR). It is thought that NLR can predict prognosis, due to its close relationship with the cancer stage [3,7,9,10]. Increased preoperative NLR is caused by neutrophilia and/or lymphopenia, the two conditions of a pro-tumor inflammatory process. This value is, however, questioned because an elevated number of neutrophils indicates an acute SIR, whereas, cancers cause chronic SIR [5,11].

Chronic SIR is thought to be estimated by the LMR value [5]. In rectal cancer, in contrast to previously reported findings with NLR, it was observed that the preoperative LMR values were lower in patients with large tumors diagnosed in late stages [12]. Preoperative serum parameters are important for establishing treatment strategies [5]. Large cohorts are needed to establish the reliability of these cheap and easily quantified markers.

The present study aimed to validate the possible prognostic or predictive impact of preoperative NLR and LMR in a large cohort of patients with rectal cancer. The included patients underwent surgery in two university surgical departments, one from Romania and one from Hungary.

2. Materials and Methods

2.1. Patient Selection

The approval of the three Ethical Committees (Ethical Committee of the Clinical County Emergency Hospital and the Ethical Committee of the George Emil Palade University of Medicine, Pharmacy, Sciences and Technology, Targu Mures, Romania; Institutional Research Ethics Committee from Budapest, Hungary) was obtained for this study.

We performed a retrospective observational study that included all consecutive patients with rectal cancer who underwent surgery, between January 2013 and August 2019, in two university hospitals: The National Institute of Oncology of Budapest, Hungary, and the Emergency Clinical County Hospital of Targu Mures, Romania.

Besides preoperative serum values of NLR and LMR ratio, the following clinicopathological parameters were examined: Patient's gender and age, the type of surgical procedure (with or without sphincter preservation), presence or absence of preoperative chemoradiotherapy (CRT), and tumor location (low vs. mid/upper rectum), along with the pTNM stage and overall survival rate (OS) rate. Patient follow-up ranged from 1 to 76 months.

Most of the patients received capecitabine/long-course radiation therapy or 5-fluorouracil (5-FU)/long-course radiation therapy (50 Gy in 28 fractions). Blood analyses were done one day before the surgical intervention or early in the morning on the day of surgery. To allow patient recuperation, an interval of 6–8 weeks passed between CRT and surgery.

The surgical approaches were abdominal-perineal excision of the rectum (APER), anterior resection (Dixon), and Hartmann's resection. These interventions were performed by two highly experienced surgical teams in the two clinical centers.

The pathologists evaluated the macroscopical quality of total mesorectal excision (TME), which was scored as complete, partially complete, and incomplete. They also performed the microscopic evaluation of the depth of infiltration (pT stage), the quality of resection margins, the lymph node status (pN stage), and lymph node ratio (LNR) and established the pTNM stage [4].

Our study included patients over 18 years old, diagnosed with rectal cancer, with or without CRT, with preoperatively defined NLR and LMR, who underwent laparoscopic or open surgery.

Exclusion criteria included biopsies, cases where death occurred less than one month postoperatively, patients with associated sepsis, autoimmune or hematologic diseases, and cases with incomplete available information.

2.2. Statistical Analysis

Data analysis was performed using Graph Pad Prism 7 and SPSS software. Nominal variables were characterized using frequencies. Quantitative variables were tested for normality of distribution using the Kolmogorov-Smirnov test and were characterized by median and percentiles (25th–75th) or by the mean and standard deviation (SD), as appropriate.

We used the Chi-squared test, Student's t-test, Mann Whitney test, and Spearman correlation test. We used the cut-off value of 3.11 for NLR and 3.39 for LMR, respectively. The cut-off values were defined according to TME quality (1 was considered complete, and 0 was considered partially complete or incomplete). A receiver-operating characteristic (ROC) curve analysis was used to test the predictive power and to determine cut-off values for NLR and LMR. We estimated the OS using the Kaplan-Meier curves; log-rank tests were applied for pair-wise comparison of survival. To distinguish non-significant cofactors from significant independent predictors of OS, multivariate Cox proportional hazards regression analyses and backward stepwise elimination were used. The Cox model was adjusted for age, gender, pTNM stage, lymph node ratio (LNR), and distal resection margin quality. All tests were two-tailed tests, and a *p*-value < 0.05 was considered statistically significant.

3. Results

3.1. Clinicopathological Parameters

We retrospectively evaluated a database of 1052 patients with rectal cancer diagnosed over six years. Included patients had a mean age of 64.29 ± 11.32 (range 21–94) years. There was a male predominance, with 61.9% males and 38.1% females (M:F ratio was 1.62:1).

In three-quarters of the patients (74.8%), the tumor involved the middle/upper rectum (which encompassed an area 5–15 cm). The ratio between middle/upper and lower (<5 cm) rectum involvement was 2.96:1. As a consequence, sphincter-preserving surgery was done in 70.5% of patients; with a ratio of 2.39:1 (preserving vs. non-preserving sphincter). The ratio between the node-negative and node-positive cases was 1.39:1. A ratio of 2.20:1 was observed between locally advanced stages (pT3-4) and cases with a low level of infiltration (pT1-2) (Table 1).

Table 1. Correlation between clinicopathological factors and serum indicators of systemic inflammatory response.

Clinicopathological Parameters		Number n = 1052 (%)	NLR			LMR		
			<3.11 (23.9%)	≥3.11 (76.1%)	*p* Value	<3.39 (82.0%)	≥3.39 (18.0%)	*p* Value *
Gender	Male	(61.9)	(56.1)	(63.7)	0.05	(64.6)	(50.0)	0.001
	Female	(38.1)	(43.9)	(36.3)		(35.4)	(50.0)	
Age (years)	<60	(30.8)	(26.0)	(32.3)	0.09	(30.8)	(30.4)	0.92
	≥60	(69.2)	(74.0)	(67.7)		(69.2)	(69.6)	
Tumor location	Low	(25.2)	(14.8)	(27.0)	0.01	(28.2)	(7.7)	0.0001
	Mid/upper	(74.8)	(85.2)	(73.0)		(71.8)	(92.3)	
Depth of infiltration	pT1-2	(31.2)	(28.2)	(32.2)	0.30	(32.7)	(24.3)	0.05
	pT3-4	(68.8)	(71.8)	(67.8)		(67.3)	(75.7)	
Lymph node status	pN0	(58.2)	(60.0)	(50.0)	0.02	(60.0)	(50.0)	0.02
	pN+	(41.8)	(40.0)	(50.0)		(40.0)	(50.0)	
Sphincter-preserving	Yes	(70.5)	(83.2)	(66.6)	0.0001	(67.9)	(82.4)	0.0001
	No	(29.5)	(16.8)	(33.4)		(32.1)	(17.6)	
Preoperative oncologic therapy	Yes	(62.0)	(30.6)	(71.8)	0.0001	(68.0)	(34.5)	0.0001
	No	(38.0)	(69.4)	(28.2)		(32.0)	(65.5)	

(NLR = neutrophil-to-lymphocyte ratio; LMR = lymphocyte-to-monocyte ratio; * Chi square test).

The average time of the surgical interventions was 145 min. The laparoscopic surgeries required a significantly longer time ($p < 0.0001$), compared to the open interventions (162 vs. 128 min), without improving OS ($p = 0.44$) (Figure 1). However, significantly longer hospitalization was needed for patients who underwent open surgical intervention. Patients spent an average of two additional days in the hospital, compared with patients who underwent a laparoscopic intervention ($p = 0.004$). A significant difference was observed between open and laparoscopic approaches in the timing of the patient's first stool in the postoperative period ($p < 0.0001$). The first stool was present one day earlier after laparoscopic interventions than after open surgery.

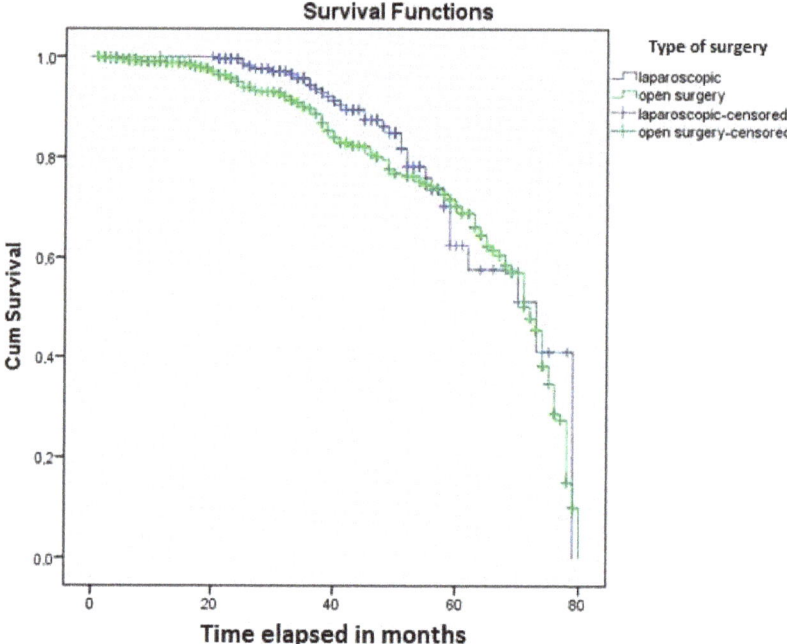

Figure 1. Patients with rectal cancer who underwent laparoscopic surgery did not show a longer overall survival than those who were treated by open surgery ($p = 0.44$).

3.2. Particularities of the Systemic Inflammatory Response

An inverse correlation between LMR and NLR values was observed ($p < 0.0001$). This correlation was also highlighted when we compared the LMR and NLR values in males vs. females. Comparing with females, male patients showed slightly higher NLR and lower LMR values, independently by the patient's age, especially for the cases of lower rectum who received preoperative CRT (Table 1).

As regarding NLR, independently from the depth of tumor infiltration, the NLR values were slightly lower in patients with tumors of the mid/upper rectum who did not show lymph node metastases and were treated with sphincter preserving, before receiving CRT (Table 1). Furthermore, there was no significant association between the clinical TNM tumor stage and NLR or LMR ($p = 0.30$, $p = 0.06$, respectively). LNR was not influenced by NLR ($p = 0.13$), but was associated with LMR value ($p = 0.03$).

A significant association was observed between the tumor distance from the anal verge and NLR ($p < 0.0001$) or LMR value ($p < 0.0001$), indicating that a longer distance from the anal margin results in a lower NLR and a higher LMR. The distance from the anal verge was directly associated with the tumor stage ($p = 0.006$). The lower rectum tumors presented mainly lower stages, while tumor perforation was more common when the tumor was localized at the upper level ($p = 0.01$). When CRT was initiated, the incidence of tumor perforation decreased considerably ($p = 0.01$). However, independent of tumor location (low vs. mid/upper rectum), a considerable number of cases (83.2%) from the low NLR group underwent sphincter-preserving surgery, in contrast with the high NLR group, where this rate was only 66.6% (Table 1).

LMR values were lower in patients with cancers of the lower rectum who responded to preoperative CRT and did not show lymph node metastases or deep infiltration (pT1-2N0 cases). In these patients, sphincter preservation was not frequently the therapy of choice (Table 1).

The integrity of the mesorectum following TME was significantly associated with the LMR ($p = 0.0009$), and the NLR value ($p = 0.0005$), same as with the total number of harvested lymph nodes ($p = 0.01$) and LNR ($p = 0.04$). In cases with higher NLR values, the integrity of the mesorectum was only partially complete or incomplete, reflecting an abundant tissue inflammation. In these cases, the value of the NLR did not significantly correlate with the duration of the surgery ($p = 0.18$, $r = 0.06$), although the surgery time was associated with the TME quality.

In those cases that required a shorter time of surgery, the TME was more frequently complete ($p = 0.01$), in contrast with difficult cases, which demanded a longer time. Obviously, TME quality was significantly associated with the tumor invasion of the circumferential resection margin invasion ($p < 0.0001$).

The above-mentioned correlations and associations showed that an NLR value of ≥ 3.11 can be used to indicate the response to preoperative CRT, but a low chance of sphincter preservation or obtaining a complete TME. Based on the same algorithm, an LMR value of ≥ 3.39 might indicate deep invasion or absence of preoperative CRT (Table 1).

3.3. Overall Survival

The Kaplan-Meier analysis showed a significant influence of neoadjuvant treatment on patients' OS ($p = 0.0001$) (Figure 2). OS was found to be significantly influenced by SIR, defined by the cut-off values for NLR ($p = 0.03$) (Figure 3) and LMR ($p = 0.04$) (Figure 4).

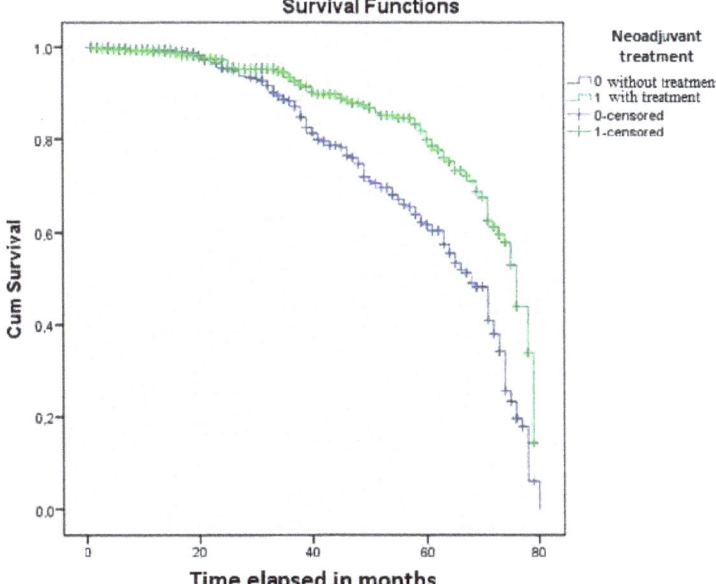

Figure 2. Neoadjuvant treatment significantly influences patients' survival rate, compared to those who did not receive preoperative oncotherapy ($p = 0.0001$).

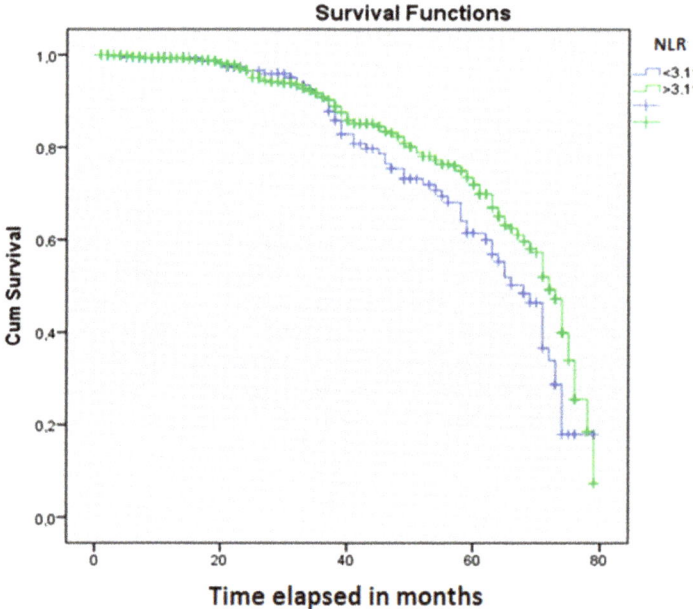

Figure 3. The cut-off value of 3.11 for the NLR can be used as an independent prognostic parameter for patients with rectal cancer ($p = 0.03$).

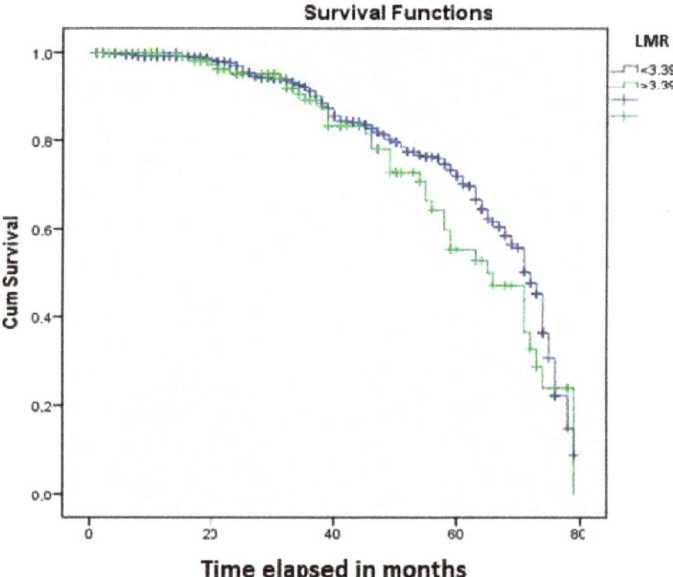

Figure 4. The cut-off value of 3.39 for the LMR can be used as an independent prognostic parameter for patients with rectal cancer ($p = 0.04$).

Other parameters which significantly influenced patients' survival rate were age group ($p = 0.04$) and gender ($p = 0.007$, male patients live longer), TNM stage ($p < 0.0001$), LNR ($p < 0.0001$), positivity of the distal resection margin ($p < 0.0001$), and tumor perforation ($p < 0.0001$). There was no statistically significant correlation between OS and tumor distance from the anal margin ($p = 0.52$).

4. Discussion

The immune response and SIR influence the rate of tumor growth and the risk of metastasis [3]. Strong tumor infiltration by inflammatory cells (including neutrophils) may contribute to intensified proliferation and tumor angiogenesis [4,9,12–14]. In these cases, the response to CRT may be altered [4].

As defined, the NLR is the ratio between the absolute number of neutrophils and the absolute number of lymphocytes [4,15]. Furthermore, LMR represents the absolute number of lymphocytes divided by the absolute number of monocytes [11]. Regarding NLR, an antitumor immunity suppressing role is attributed to neutrophils [15]. This suppression contributes to cancer progression, which is augmented by lymphocytopenia [3,14]. In contrast, high levels of tumor-infiltrating lymphocytes (TIL) are correlated with a longer OS [3,12]. This is attributed to cytotoxic activity and anti-angiogenetic cytokine production [4,11].

Although the investigated parameters (NLR, LMR) might be associated with the tumor stage, the literature data are controversial, and the underlying mechanisms of these results are not fully elucidated. For this reason, these ratios cannot yet consider independent prognostic factors [11,16]. They are influenced by several factors, which should be considered. Moreover, due to the behavior, anatomical topography, and therapeutic management of rectal cancer, the rate of inflammatory markers could have different relevance [13,17]. For example, an increased LMR might be induced by autoimmune or hematologic diseases, but also by infections [9], aspects that can explain the higher rate of incomplete TME in the cases with LMR ≥3.39.

The NLR and LMR values might also be influenced by preoperative CRT. Abe et al. demonstrated lower values for LMR in patients with tumors diagnosed in pT1-2N0 stages, in patients with rectal cancer who did not receive preoperative CRT, without correlation of LMR with tumor stage, after CRT [5]. Other authors, such as Caputo et al., have demonstrated no correlation with tumor stage [4], with a negative impact on OS [8,18] or, contrary, no impact of LMR on OS or disease-free survival [19]. Our apparently contradictory results, which proved at the limit of statistical significance ($p = 0.05$), lower LMR values for pT1-2N0 cases, are in line with data reported by authors, such as Mallapa et al. [16] or Abe et al. [5]. We did not find an association of LMR with LNR, which was defined as the number of positive lymph nodes divided by the total number of lymph nodes harvested [20,21], and not reported to the rectal lymph nodes only.

The controversial literature reports might be explained based on the number of examined cases (usually below 300), the used protocols therapeutically and the homogeneity of the cohort. As most of the authors perform statistical examinations in consecutive cases and establish "in-house" managed ratios, using receiver operating curve analysis [8], such in our material, controversial data might be influenced by these above-mentioned factors. It is necessary to mention, for example, that 68.8% of patients included in the present study were diagnosed in patients with pT3/4 staged tumors, with or without lymph node metastases, and correlations were done based on the cut-off value of 3.39. In contrast with other authors [7,16], we have included in the examined databases only rectal carcinomas, without tumors located in the colon or in the anal canal. On the other hand, some authors, such as Xiao et al. included only patients in the pT3N0 stage [18].

In patients with CRC, poorer OS was predicted when pre-treatment NLR showed elevated values [22]. In our material, the applied cut-off value for NLR was 3.11. An NLR of >3, before CRT/before surgery, is usually considered an indicator of poor prognosis, high recurrence rate, and low 5-year OS [4,15,23]. As regarding tumor stage, Caputo et al. reported, similar to our data, no significant association between the pTNM stage and NLR [4]. A higher clinical stage III rate was observed by Cha et al. in their cases within high NLR [11]. Other authors reported increased NLR in cases with positive nodal status on MRI [13,14]—this latter aspect being also proved by our data. Based on an in-house evaluation of large cohorts, a cut-off value should be established for prognostic evaluation [24,25]. In our material, NLR ≥3.11 and LMR <3.39 proved to be indicators of the response to preoperative CRT and lower risk for lymph node metastases.

Regarding TME, its quality was more frequent incomplete or only partially complete in cases with high NLR values. This aspect can be related to the surgical intervention quality or can reflect a peritumoral extensive inflammatory profile, which does not allow a proper and complete mesorectal excision. Scarce data can be found in the literature about the possible relationship between NLR and TME quality. Authors, such as Sung et al. [26] or Portal et al. [10], agree with the idea that pre-CRT and post-CRT NLR value might be used as a blood biomarker with a potential prognostic role in the case of patients who underwent curative TME intervention [10,26], but we did not find other supplementary explanation for this relationship. However, a high NLR and a low LMR value will lead in the majority of the cases to an incomplete TME quality, which will negatively influence patient's OS, disease-free survival, and recurrence survival. In these circumstances, surgeons can identify preoperatively patients with a high risk of developing postoperative complications [4,27,28].

The strength of the present study consists of the investigation of one of the largest sample sizes so far, including only rectal cancer cases, from two medical centers. The limitations consist of its retrospective manner, and of including only two surgical centers, with predominantly locally advanced cases. These limitations were mitigated by using the largest databases reported in the literature, establishing an in-house designed value for both NLR and LMR. To elucidate the possible geographic-related differences, also reported for other cancers [29], a further multicenter study, in a larger cohort, should be performed.

5. Conclusions

The investigated parameters, NLR and LMR, are useful independent prognostic parameters. An NLR value of ≥3.11 can be used to indicate the response to preoperative CRT, but a low chance of sphincter preservation or obtaining a complete TME. An LMR value of ≥3.39 might indicate deep tumor invasion. The fact that NLR and LMR seem to influence the TME integrity is of great importance, which should be considered by rectal surgeons.

Author Contributions: Conceptualization, S.G. and Z.Z.F.; data curation, Z.Z.F. and J.T.; formal analysis, Z.Z.F. and R.L.F.; investigation, R.L.F., T.B.J. and E.D.; methodology, R.L.F., T.B.J. and I.J.; project administration, S.G.; resources, J.T.; software, E.D.; supervision, I.J.; validation, E.D.; visualization, E.D.; Writing—review & editing, J.T. and I.J.; Z.Z.F. and R.L.F. have equal contribution to the paper. All authors have read and agreed to the published version of the manuscript.

Funding: This research was funded by the Collegium Talentum 2019 Program of Hungary (research bursary for first author) and a grant of the Romanian National Authority for Scientific Research, CNCS—UEFISCDI, project number 20 PCCF/2018, code: PN-III-P4-ID-PCCF-2016-0006. The APC was funded by GE Palade University of Medicine, Pharmacy, Sciences and Technology, Targu-Mures, Romania.

Acknowledgments: The authors would like to express their sincere gratitude for the Hungarian team from the National Institute of Oncology, namely Mersich Tamás, Head of the Visceral Surgery Department, Gödény Mária, Head of the Radiology Department and Strausz Tamás from the Pathology Department. We also thank to our colleagues from Clinical County Emergency Hospital of Targu-Mues, Romania, for their help in treating patients and performing their follow-up and to Septimiu Voidăzan for statistical assessment.

Conflicts of Interest: The authors declare no conflict of interest.

References

1. Dekker, E.; Tanis, P.J.; Vleugels, J.L.A.; Kasi, P.M.; Wallace, M.B. Colorectal cancer. *Lancet* **2019**, *394*, 1467–1480. [CrossRef]
2. Tamas, K.; Walenkamp, A.M.E.; De Vries, E.G.E.; Van Vugt, M.A.T.M.; Beets-Tan, R.G.; Van Etten, B.; De Groot, D.J.A.; Hospers, G.A.P. Rectal and colon cancer: Not just a different anatomic site. *Cancer Treat. Rev.* **2015**, *41*, 671–679. [CrossRef] [PubMed]

3. Yoshida, D.; Minami, K.; Sugiyama, M.; Ota, M.; Ikebe, M.; Morita, M.; Matsukuma, A.; Toh, Y. Prognostic Impact of the Neutrophil-to-Lymphocyte Ratio in Stage I-II Rectal Cancer Patients. *J. Surg. Res.* **2019**, *245*, 281–287. [CrossRef] [PubMed]
4. Caputo, D.; Caricato, M.; Coppola, A.; La Vaccara, V.; Fiore, M.; Coppola, R. Neutrophil to Lymphocyte Ratio (NLR) and Derived Neutrophil to Lymphocyte Ratio (d-NLR) Predict Non-Responders and Postoperative Complications in Patients Undergoing Radical Surgery After Neo-Adjuvant Radio-Chemotherapy for Rectal Adenocarcinoma. *Cancer Investig.* **2016**, *34*, 440–451. [CrossRef] [PubMed]
5. Abe, S.; Kawai, K.; Nozawa, H.; Hata, K.; Kiyomatsu, T.; Morikawa, T.; Watanabe, T. LMR predicts outcome in patients after preoperative chemoradiotherapy for stage II-III rectal cancer. *J. Surg. Res.* **2018**, *222*, 122–131. [CrossRef] [PubMed]
6. Su, P.-Z.; Dong, Y.-W.; Shi, Y.-Q.; He, L.-W. Prognostic significance of neutrophil-to-lymphocyte ratio in rectal cancer: A meta-analysis. *OncoTargets Ther.* **2016**, *9*, 3127–3134. [CrossRef]
7. De Felice, F.; Rubini, F.L.; Romano, L.; Bulzonetti, N.; Caiazzo, R.; Musio, D.; Tombolini, V. Prognostic significance of inflammatory-related parameters in patients with anal canal cancer. *Int. J. Colorectal Dis.* **2019**, *34*, 519–525. [CrossRef]
8. Deng, Y.-X.; Lin, J.-Z.; Peng, J.-H.; Zhao, Y.-J.; Sui, Q.-Q.; Wu, X.-J.; Lu, Z.-H.; Gao, Y.-H.; Zeng, Z.-F.; Pan, Z.-Z. Lymphocyte-to-monocyte ratio before chemoradiotherapy represents a prognostic predictor for locally advanced rectal cancer. *OncoTargets Ther.* **2017**, *10*, 5575–5583. [CrossRef]
9. Chiang, S.-F.; Hung, H.-Y.; Tang, R.; Changchien, C.R.; Chen, J.-S.; You, Y.-T.; Chiang, J.-M.; Lin, J.-R. Can neutrophil-to-lymphocyte ratio predict the survival of colorectal cancer patients who have received curative surgery electively? *Int. J. Colorectal Dis.* **2012**, *27*, 1347–1357. [CrossRef]
10. Portale, G.; Cavallin, F.; Valdegamberi, A.; Frigo, F.; Fiscon, V. Platelet-to-Lymphocyte Ratio and Neutrophil-to-Lymphocyte Ratio Are Not Prognostic Biomarkers in Rectal Cancer Patients with Curative Resection. *J. Gastrointest. Surg.* **2018**, *22*, 1611–1618. [CrossRef]
11. Cha, Y.J.; Park, E.J.; Baik, S.H.; Lee, K.Y.; Kang, J. Prognostic impact of persistent lower neutrophil-to-lymphocyte ratio during preoperative chemoradiotherapy in locally advanced rectal cancer patients: A propensity score matching analysis. *PLoS ONE* **2019**, *14*, e0214415. [CrossRef] [PubMed]
12. Braun, L.H.; Baumann, D.; Clasen, K.; Eipper, E.; Hauth, F.; Peter, A.; Zips, D.; Gani, C. Neutrophil-to-Lymphocyte Ratio in Rectal Cancer-Novel Biomarker of Tumor Immunogenicity During Radiotherapy or Confounding Variable? *Int. J. Mol. Sci.* **2019**, *20*, 2448. [CrossRef]
13. Khan, A.A.; Akritidis, G.; Pring, T.; Alagaratnam, S.; Roberts, G.; Raymond, R.; Varcada, M.; Novell, R. The Neutrophil-to-Lymphocyte Ratio as a Marker of Lymph Node Status in Patients with Rectal Cancer. *Oncology* **2016**, *91*, 69–77. [CrossRef]
14. Li, H.; Song, J.; Cao, M.; Wang, G.; Li, L.-T.; Zhang, B.; Li, Y.; Xu, W.; Zheng, J. Preoperative neutrophil-to-lymphocyte ratio is a more valuable prognostic factor than platelet-to-lymphocyte ratio for nonmetastatic rectal cancer. *Int. Immunopharmacol.* **2016**, *40*, 327–331. [CrossRef]
15. Howard, R.; Kanetsky, P.A.; Egan, K.M. Exploring the prognostic value of the neutrophil-to-lymphocyte ratio in cancer. *Sci. Rep.* **2019**, *9*, 19673. [CrossRef] [PubMed]
16. Mallappa, S.; Sinha, A.; Gupta, S.; Chadwick, S.J.D. Preoperative neutrophil to lymphocyte ratio >5 is a prognostic factor for recurrent colorectal cancer. *Colorectal Dis.* **2013**, *15*, 323–328. [CrossRef]
17. Banias, L.; Jung, I.; Bara, T.; Fulop, Z.; Simu, P.; Simu, I.; Satala, C.; Gurzu, S. Immunohistochemical-based molecular subtyping of colorectal carcinoma using maspin and markers of epithelial-mesenchymal transition. *Oncol. Lett.* **2019**, *19*, 1487–1495. [CrossRef]
18. Xiao, W.-W.; Zhang, L.-N.; You, K.-Y.; Huang, R.; Yu, X.; Ding, P.-R.; Gao, Y.-H. A Low Lymphocyte-to-Monocyte Ratio Predicts Unfavorable Prognosis in Pathological T3N0 Rectal Cancer Patients Following Total Mesorectal Excision. *J. Cancer* **2015**, *6*, 616–622. [CrossRef] [PubMed]
19. Wu, Q.-B.; Wang, M.; Hu, T.; He, W.-B.; Wang, Z.-Q. Prognostic role of the lymphocyte-to-monocyte ratio in patients undergoing resection for nonmetastatic rectal cancer. *Medicine (Baltimore)* **2016**, *95*, e4945. [CrossRef]
20. Fulop, Z.Z.; Gurzu, S.; Dragus, E.; Bara, T.; Voidazan, S.; Banias, L.; Jung, I. Lymph node ratio, an independent prognostic factor for patients with stage II-III rectal carcinoma. *Pathol. Res. Pract.* **2019**, *215*, 152384. [CrossRef]

21. Molnar, C.; Nicolescu, C.; Grigorescu, B.L.; Botoncea, M.; Butiurca, V.O.; Petrisor, M.; Gurzu, S. Comparative oncological outcomes and survival following surgery for low rectal cancer—A single center experience. *Rom. J. Morphol. Embryol.* **2019**, *60*, 847–852. [PubMed]
22. Li, M.-X.; Liu, X.; Zhang, X.-F.; Zhang, J.-F.; Wang, W.-L.; Zhu, Y.; Dong, J.; Cheng, J.-W.; Liu, Z.; Ma, L.; et al. Prognostic role of neutrophil-to-lymphocyte ratio in colorectal cancer: A systematic review and meta-analysis. *Int. J. Cancer* **2014**, *134*, 2403–2413. [CrossRef] [PubMed]
23. Nagasaki, T.; Akiyoshi, T.; Fujimoto, Y.; Konishi, T.; Nagayama, S.; Fukunaga, Y.; Ueno, M. Prognostic Impact of Neutrophil-to-Lymphocyte Ratio in Patients with Advanced Low Rectal Cancer Treated with Preoperative Chemoradiotherapy. *Dig. Surg.* **2015**, *32*, 496–503. [CrossRef] [PubMed]
24. Haram, A.; Boland, M.R.; Kelly, M.E.; Bolger, J.C.; Waldron, R.M.; Kerin, M.J. The prognostic value of neutrophil-to-lymphocyte ratio in colorectal cancer: A systematic review. *J. Surg. Oncol.* **2017**, *115*, 470–479. [CrossRef]
25. Gani, C.; Bonomo, P.; Zwirner, K.; Schroeder, C.; Menegakis, A.; Rödel, C.; Zips, D. Organ preservation in rectal cancer—Challenges and future strategies. *Clin. Transl. Radiat. Oncol.* **2017**, *3*, 9–15. [CrossRef]
26. Sung, S.; Son, S.H.; Park, E.Y.; Kay, C.S. Prognosis of locally advanced rectal cancer can be predicted more accurately using pre- and post-chemoradiotherapy neutrophil-lymphocyte ratios in patients who received preoperative chemoradiotherapy. *PLoS ONE* **2017**, *12*, e0173955. [CrossRef]
27. Lino-Silva, L.S.; SalcedoHernndez, R.; RuizGarca, E.; HerreraGmez, L.; Salcedo-Hernández, R.A.; Ruíz-García, E.; García-Pérez, L.; Herrera-Gómez, Á. Pre-operative Neutrophils/Lymphocyte Ratio in Rectal Cancer Patients with Preoperative Chemoradiotherapy. *Med. Arch.* **2016**, *70*, 256–260. [CrossRef]
28. Jung, S.W.; Oh, S.G.; Oh, S.H.; Yeom, S.-S.; Lee, J.L.; Yoon, Y.S.; Kim, C.W.; Lim, S.-B.; Lee, J.B.; Yu, C.S.; et al. Association of immunologic markers from complete blood counts with the response to preoperative chemoradiotherapy and prognosis in locally advanced rectal cancer. *Oncotarget* **2017**, *8*, 59757–59765. [CrossRef]
29. Kádár, Z.; Jung, I.; Orlowska, J.; Szentirmay, Z.; Sugimura, H.; Turdean, S.; Simona, G. Geographic particularities in incidence and etiopathogenesis of sporadic gastric cancer. *Pol. J. Pathol.* **2015**, *3*, 254–259. [CrossRef]

Publisher's Note: MDPI stays neutral with regard to jurisdictional claims in published maps and institutional affiliations.

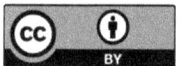

© 2020 by the authors. Licensee MDPI, Basel, Switzerland. This article is an open access article distributed under the terms and conditions of the Creative Commons Attribution (CC BY) license (http://creativecommons.org/licenses/by/4.0/).

Review

Predictive Biomarkers of Oxaliplatin-Induced Peripheral Neurotoxicity

Roser Velasco [1,2,*], Montserrat Alemany [1], Macarena Villagrán [1] and Andreas A. Argyriou [3]

1. Neurology Department, Neuro-Oncology Unit-IDIBELL, Hospital Universitari de Bellvitge-Institut Català d'Oncologia L'Hospitalet, 08907 Barcelona, Spain; malemany@bellvitgehospital.cat (M.A.); mac.vgarcia@gmail.com (M.V.)
2. Institute of Neurosciences, Department of Cell Biology, Physiology and Immunology, Universitat Autònoma de Barcelona, and Centro de Investigación Biomédica en Red sobre Enfermedades Neurodegenerativas (CIBERNED), 08193 Bellaterra, Spain
3. Neurology Department, "Saint Andrew's" State General Hospital of Patras, 26335 Patras, Greece; andargyriou@yahoo.gr
* Correspondence: rvelascof@bellvitgehospital.cat; Tel.: +34-932607500

Abstract: Oxaliplatin (OXA) is a platinum compound primarily used in the treatment of gastrointestinal cancer. OXA-induced peripheral neurotoxicity (OXAIPN) is the major non-hematological dose-limiting toxicity of OXA-based chemotherapy and includes acute transient neurotoxic effects that appear soon after OXA infusion, and chronic non-length dependent sensory neuronopathy symmetrically affecting both upper and lower limbs in a stocking-and-glove distribution. No effective strategy has been established to reverse or treat OXAIPN. Thus, it is necessary to early predict the occurrence of OXAIPN during treatment and possibly modify the OXA-based regimen in patients at high risk as an early diagnosis and intervention may slow down neuropathy progression. However, identifying which patients are more likely to develop OXAIPN is clinically challenging. Several objective and measurable early biomarkers for OXAIPN prediction have been described in recent years, becoming useful for informing clinical decisions about treatment. The purpose of this review is to critically review data on currently available or promising predictors of OXAIPN. Neurological monitoring, according to predictive factors for increased risk of OXAIPN, would allow clinicians to personalize treatment, by monitoring at-risk patients more closely and guide clinicians towards better counseling of patients about neurotoxicity effects of OXA.

Keywords: neurotoxicity; oxaliplatin; chemotherapy-induced peripheral neuropathy; biomarker; genomics; neuropathy; FOLFOX; FOLFIRINOX; XELOX; gastrointestinal cancer

1. Introduction

Oxaliplatin (OXA) is widely used for the treatment of gastrointestinal cancers including colorectal (CRC), gastric, and pancreatic cancer, both in the adjuvant and metastatic setting [1,2]. OXA-induced peripheral neurotoxicity (OXAIPN) is the major non-hematological cause for dose-reduction as also discontinuation of OXA-based chemotherapy and it is manifested with two clinically distinct forms. The acute, neuromyotonia-like syndrome, as a result of hyperexcited sensory and motor nerves, appears soon after OXA, is transient and usually completely reversible within hours or days [3]. Patients may also develop chronic sensory symmetrical symptoms, including tingling, numbness and pain in a 'stocking/glove' distribution developing during treatment, while up to 20% of patients can be severely affected to develop sensory ataxia and increased susceptibility to falls [4–6]. Five years after finishing chemotherapy, 25–30% of patients suffer from clinically significant chronic OXAIPN [3,7], without modification in this rate over 3–8 years [8–11]. Persistent OXAIPN is associated with psychological distress, depression and impaired quality of life in long-term gastrointestinal cancer survivors [8].

Given the lack of effective symptomatic or preventive treatment strategies against both acute and chronic OXAIPN [9], in daily practice, neurological symptoms referred by patients are usually taken into account to adapt OXA dosing in order to prevent severe neuropathy (Figure 1). Treating physician will indicate dose adjustment of OXA administering significantly less cumulative than planned doses of anti-cancer treatment what may compromise patient survival [10], therefore becoming a critical decision balancing the maximization of therapeutic benefit and the minimization of this significant OXA toxicity. Importantly, the observed worsening of OXAIPN weeks after cessation of treatment complicates clinical decisions regarding the duration and total dose of OXA in individual patients based on symptoms of sensory neuropathy alone.

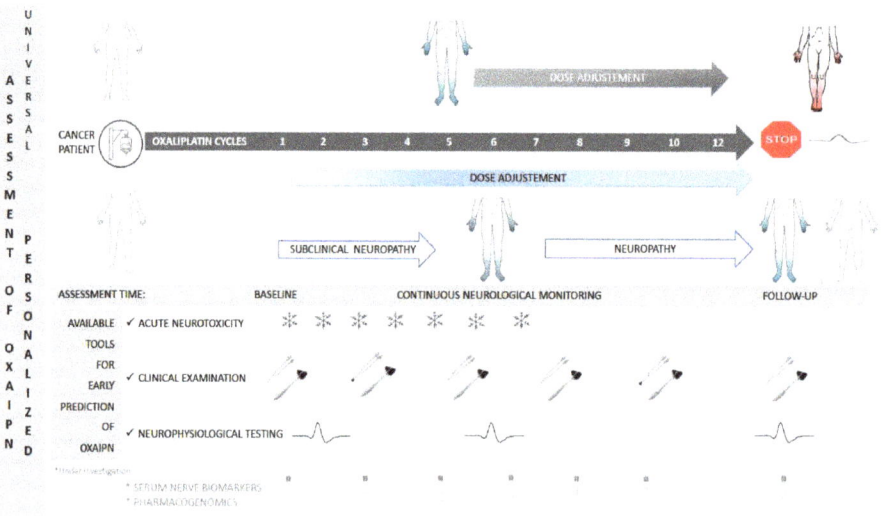

Figure 1. Personalized assessment of neuropathy by present and future strategies to early detecting and monitoring oxaliplatin-induced peripheral neuropathy in gastrointestinal cancer patients.

Cumulative dose of OXA is the main predictor of OXAIPN [12–14], with increasing rates from 42.5% to 76.7% with median cumulative dose of ≤ 780 mg/m^2 and >780 mg/m^2, respectively [11], also when re-challenging patients with OXA in further lines [15,16]. However, the relationship between dose and neurotoxicity might not be linear before reaching a cumulative dose level beyond which the toxicity becomes dose-dependent [17]. OXAIPN development cannot be accurately predicted in a gastrointestinal cancer patient before OXA treatment initiation and the common inter-individual variability in severity of OXAIPN in the setting of a uniform insult is a major challenge in clinical practice. Early prediction of development and progression of OXAIPN and a timely decision to decrease the OXA dosing in patients at high risk is clinically important. In recent years, several clinical and neurophysiological predictive biomarkers that can be easily obtained before or early during treatment to estimate which patients are at higher risk for OXAIPN have been described. From the personalized medicine perspective, having non-invasive, sensitive and specific biomarkers, will allow patients more liable to OXAIPN to prevent the occurrence of long-term toxicity or permanent damage. These objective markers may aid in the prediction of the development, severity and duration OXAIPN, and in adjusting OXA dose more precisely to balance the risk of neurotoxicity against antineoplastic efficacy. This review focuses on the currently available biomarkers of early OXAIPN detection that may allow clinicians to closely monitor at-risk patients and personalize treatment according to neurotoxicity risk of OXA.

2. Clinical Factors Associated with OXAIPN

2.1. Pre-Treatment Factors

A variety of pretreatment patient- or environmental-related risks have been described in the literature with conflicting results (Table 1). Methodological issues, such as the relatively small size, the retrospective design and the lack of statistical approach with multivariate regression analysis in many of them, likely underly limitations in the generalization of available results. To date, no demographic factors or preexisting comorbidities including age, diabetes mellitus or preexisting neuropathy have been consistently identified across multiple studies helpful in the prediction of the development, severity or duration of OXAIPN [18] that should be considered for upfront screening in a priori patients' risk classification.

Table 1. Factors investigated that are or not associated with the incidence and severity of oxaliplatin induced peripheral neurotoxicity.

Variable at Baseline	Associated	Not Associated
Age	[12] * [14,15,19] * [13,16]	[20,21] [22,23] *
Gender	[24]	[12,15,22] * [20,23,25]
BSA (Body Surface Area)	[12] * [13]	[23,26]
BMI (Body Mass Index)	[27,28]	[12,14,19,29] *
Body Weight	[12] *	[19] * [26]
Concurrent treatments	[12,30] * [31]	[32]
Creatinine (renal disfunction)	[33]	[12,19] * [34–36]
Diabetes Mellitus	[28,37] [38] #	[12,15] * [38] & [27,39]
GGT	[19] *	
Hemoglobin	[14,15,19] * [22] * [27]	
Histopathology	[19] *	
Level of Albumin	[14,15,19] *	
Magnesium	[15,40] * [27]	[14] *
Preexisting Neuropathy	[41,42]	[12] *
Race	[22] *	
Season (winter)	[13,43]	[12,19,44] *
Stage of the disease	[19,23] *	[12,19] *
Schedule of chemotherapy	[45,46] [23] *	[19,44] *
Vitamin D	[19] *	

* Studies including multivariate analysis. # Shorter time to develop OXAIPN & No differences in the incidence of OXAIPN.

2.2. Acute Neurotoxicity: The Main Clinical Predictor of OXAIPN

Shortly after every OXA infusion, many patients can experience cold-triggered painful paresthesia or neuromyotonia syndrome related with a transient axonal hyperexcitability of the peripheral nerve secondary to oxalate, generated after OXA biotransformation into its active form [3]. These acute symptoms are experienced by most of patients (90%) at some point of time during treatment [18,20,22], being usually reversible within hours or days and typically is triggered or exacerbated by cold [18,21,23,47] (Table 2). Similar to persistent OXAIPN, no factors beyond dose or infusion time seem related with the risk of developing acute OXAIPN [10,21,23–28].

Table 2. Acute symptoms or signs of OXA induced neurotoxicity.

ACUTE OXALIPLATIN- INDUCED NEUROTOXICITY
Cold-induced perioral paresthesia
Cold-induced pharyngolaryngeal dysesthesia
Shortness of breath
Difficulty swallowing
Laryngospasm
Muscle cramps
Jaw stiffness
Visible fasciculations
Voice changes
Ptosis
Ocular changes

Acute neurotoxicity is a well-established risk factor for developing chronic OXAIPN at the end of chemotherapy. Clinically, several studies show that the onset and severity of acute OXAIPN is associated with the occurrence of persistent neurotoxicity [4,10,20,24,29,30]. Attal et al. showed that the duration of cold-evoked pain and intensity of neuropathic symptoms experienced during the first three cycles predicted the extent of chronic pain experienced one year later. Cold-evoked symptoms lasting four days or more after 3rd OXA cycle predicted chronic OXAIPN (OR: 22; 95% CI: 1.54–314.74; $p = 0.02$) in a comprehensive comparative prospective study including 28 cancer patients receiving OXA, mostly CRC [20]. Our group identified that the burden of acute symptoms measured when patients have completed half of the planned OXA-based treatment (mid-treatment) was independently associated with nearly double risk (OR 1.9; CI 95% 1.2 to 3.2; $p = 0.012$) of developing severe chronic OXAIPN in a prospective multicenter study including 200 CRC patients [4,24]. In this line, presence of any acute neuropathy during cycles 1–3 was associated with persistent OXAIPN (HR: 3.65 (CI 95%; 1.40–9.56) $p = 0.008$) in a retrospective analysis of 50 CRC receiving FOLFOX schedule [12].

Early onset of acute OXAIPN seems particularly predictive of long-term neurotoxicity. Pachman et al. identified that patients who experienced severe acute OXAIPN within 6 days after first OXA infusion experienced more severe neuropathy in the remaining cycles and increased incidence of chronic OXAIPN ($p < 0.001$) [48]. Particularly, hyperacute neuropathy on the first day of the first OXA cycle was found to be a hallmark of risk of OXAIPN. Up to one third (27.7%) of patients developed hyperacute neuropathy in a retrospective study including 47 CRC patients receiving OXA-based chemotherapy. Of 13 patients who experienced hyperacute neuropathy, 12 (92.3%) eventually developed persistent OXAIPN. Multivariate analysis including the total dose of OXA and the presence of hyperacute neuropathy demonstrated that these two variables independently predicted OXAIPN [49]. The role of a such early clinical symptoms as further predictors require further validation in a in large multicenter study.

Diverse strategies have been employed for assessing acute OXA neurotoxicity. The Common Terminology Criteria for Adverse Events from the National Cancer Institute (NCI.CTC) [10,44,50], the oxaliplatin-specific neurotoxicity scale [51], or a score based on recording the frequency of symptoms with an OXA-Neuropathy Questionnaire (yes/no response format) [17,52,53], are among the most common systems for recording their presence in the daily practice. The severity of acute neurotoxicity syndrome has been defined according the burden of symptoms [54], or according to a visual analogical scale 0 (no problem) to 10 (major problem) numerical rating scale for any of the four acute neuropathy symptoms [48,55,56]. More sophisticated techniques to objectively assess acute syndrome are described below in detail.

Importantly, gastrointestinal cancer patients receiving OXA must be specifically interviewed about the presence of typical and atypical neuropathic symptoms, either these are transient or persistent. For example, recognition of acute atypical forms of OXAIPN requires a prolonged OXA infusion rate from 2 to 4 or 6 h in order to reduce risk of persistent

OXAIPN [3,57]. The implementation of a simple standardized assessment tool to monitor acute neurotoxicity in daily clinical practice should be considered due to large amount of evidence supporting the predictive role of these early manifestations in predicting persistent OXAIPN.

3. Neurophysiological and Device-Dependent Predictors

3.1. Nerve Conduction Studies (NCS) and Electromyography

Several longitudinal studies, including NCS during OXA therapy, have showed a significant progressive decrease in sensory nerve action potentials (SNAPs) and preservation of motor action compound (CMAPs), in keeping with the presence of an axonal sensory neuropathy, and consistent with the clinical symptoms and signs worsening during the treatment [17,41,58–64]. NCS are capable of objectively assessing the extent of peripheral nerve damage and may also facilitate the identification of patients that manifest subclinical peripheral neuropathy prior to the onset of clinically significant neurotoxicity. One cross-sectional study including 17 patients that had received a median of seven [8,45,65–68] treatment cycles and 850 mg/m^2 at the time of testing, disclosed that almost half of patients had evidence of sensory neuropathy. After sensory examination, reductions in upper and lower limb SNAPs of patients were the most sensitive early markers of neuropathy observed in 40% [69]. In this line, in one prospective study including 60 gastrointestinal cancer patients, sural nerve velocity and SNAP revealed a significant decrease after 50% and 100% of the planned dose, respectively [60].

NCS have also shown being useful in early predicting the neurological outcome at OXA completion. Early changes in the NCS results obtained during treatment were able to predict the development of severe OXAIPN in several prospective studies. A large multicenter study, including 200 CRC patients under treatment with FOLFOX-4, 6, and XELOX, identified at mid-treatment compared to baseline values a >30 % decrease in radial and dorsal sural SNAPs, while these abnormalities yielded a sensitivity and specificity of 96.3% and 79.1%, respectively, with positive and negative predictive values of 53% and 98.9%, for predicting severe OXAIPN at treatment completion. In the multivariate analysis, the three factors obtained at mid-treatment to independently and significantly be associated with an increased risk of severe neuropathy were: (1) having shown more symptoms of acute neurotoxicity (2) having a drop in the amplitude of the SNAP of the dorsal sural and radial nerves greater than 30%. The combination of these three factors allowed the patient with a high negative predictive value close to 99% to be classified a priori, so that in those patients with optimal NCS in the middle of treatment and who have not developed many symptoms of acute neuropathy, we could ensure with a high probability that he/she will not develop severe OXAIPN [17]. The predictiveness of dorsal sural nerve in risk stratification for OXAIPN was further evaluated in a secondary analysis of 100 CRC patients. An algorithm based on the dorsal sural nerve recordings showed that mid-treatment NCS could assign each patient to a 'neurophysiological risk class' for OXAIPN at the end of treatment [70]. In this line, reductions of the SNAPs of >11.5% in the median nerve between baseline and four cycles of OXA (odds ratio = 5.603, $p = 0.031$) and of >22.5% in the sural nerve between four and eight cycles of chemotherapy (odds ratio = 5.603, $p = 0.031$) were independently associated with the risk of developing severe OXAIPN [63]. However, very recently, negative results were obtained in another study evaluating the role of the sural nerve after administering 25% or 50% of the planned OXA dose in predicting the occurrence of clinically significant OXAIPN in 55 CRC patients [59]. The assessment of sural nerve instead dorsal sural (Figure 2), and the size of the study could underlie these negative findings. Long-term longitudinal neurophysiological assessments of OXA-treated patients have revealed a significant recovery of the SNAPs in sensory nerves in some studies [58,63,71] but not in other studies [59,61]. The length of follow-up observation may explain these differences. Unfortunately, to date, the correlation between SNAPs impairment and degree of neurotoxicity recovery remains unknown. In summary, growing evidence supports that NCS in distal sensory nerve segments offers clinicians a practical means of identifying patients more prone to severe chronic OXAIPN.

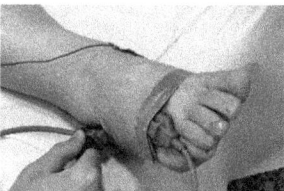

Figure 2. Nerve conduction study of the dorsal sural nerve.

Muscle sampling with needle electromyography (nEMG) can show repetitive myokymic discharges and neuromyotonic runs within 1–4 days after the first OXA administration [72–74]. However, the invasive nature of nEMG hampers its feasibility as screening tool to monitor gastrointestinal cancer patients undergoing OXA. Very recently, a simple painless objective tool to detect nerve hyperexcitability acute syndrome by a surface electromyography (sEMG) has been tested in a small study including CRC patients after the second ($n = 14$) and fourth ($n = 8$) OXA infusions revealing that sEMG is more sensitive (82%) than neurological examination (55%) to detect objective signs of acute neurotoxicity [55]. As such sEMG might be a promising test to evaluate acute oxaliplatin-induced motor nerve hyperexcitability and warrants to be further investigated in future studies.

3.2. Quantitative Sensory Tests (QST)

Quantitative sensory testing (QST) examines subjective sensory function by measuring the abnormal detection and pain thresholds to several sensory modalities. The usefulness of these non-invasive psychophysical measurements in the clinic setting for detecting subclinical neurologic changes early on to identify patients that will experience OXAIPN has been largely explored [12,20,20,42,51,53,54,56,75–82].

Vibration sensation testing can be performed by a computer controlled vibrometer or, more easily, with a tuning fork placed on a bony prominence, such as the hallux or malleollus. In both, the subject reports when they can no longer detect vibration. Impairment of the vibration detection threshold (VDT) is generally seen over the treatment course [13,20,58,61] in correlation with the progressive loss of large myelinated fibers. However, conflicting results regarding the predictive role of early changes in VDT are seen in the literature. Whereas VDT in 30 patients with gastrointestinal malignancies receiving OXA evaluated at baseline and during infusion cycles 1, 2, 4, and 6, showed no clear relationship with OXAIPN development [80], two studies including 17 [69] and 60 patients [60] showed being the earliest marker of neuropathy, present at low cumulative doses of OXA. Significant change in VDT were present after the 25% of the planed dose, being the earliest among other measures [60]. Very recently, Kroigard et al. identified VDT measure obtained before treatment correlated as a predictor of clinically significant OXAIPN six months post-treatment. However, sensitivity of a baseline VDT < 5 (maximum 8) for the prediction of clinically significant neuropathy six months after treatment was modest (76.0% (95% CI 54.9% to 90.6%)) and specificity was low (53.3% (95% CI 34.3% to 71.7%)) [59].

Mechanical detection thresholds (MDT) measures have also shown significant deterioration with increasing OXA doses in some studies [42,60] but not in others [20,82]. Touch threshold changes became statistically significant in the fingertips at middle and 8 chemotherapy doses [42] whereas these findings only occurred after treatment completion in Kroigard's study [60]. Very recently, electronic von Frey anaesthesiometer, which evaluates hyperalgesia based upon mechanical pain thresholds (MDTs), was tested prospectively in 46 CRC patients treated with OXA, and showed a decrease of 40 g in the MDT of both hands and feet as cut-off for diagnosing grade 2 or 3 OXAIPN with a total accuracy of

84.2% and 81.6% in hands and feet, respectively [78]. Besides diagnostic utility, the role MDT changes for predicting OXAIPN requires further research.

Thermal detection thresholds have been particularly investigated due to the cold-induced nature of early acute OXAIPN [79]. Attal et al. was able to detect sustained signs of neurotoxicity at an early stage when the clinical manifestations appeared to revert between OXA cycles in a comparative prospective study including 48, mainly CRC patients with who were evaluated before OXA (n = 28) or cisplatin (n = 20) and after cycles 3, 6 and 9 and after completion. Enhanced pain in response to cold (20 °C stimulus on the hand) predicted severe neuropathy (OR: 39; 95% CI: 1.8–817.8 p = 0.02) [20]. Early changes in cold (CDT) and heat detection thresholds (HDT), as predictors of clinically significant neuropathic pain six months after treatment, has been recently identified by Kroigard et al. in a prospective study including 55 patients, 14 out of them with neuropathic pain. Reduced CDT after 25% of the planned OXA dose and reduced HPT after 50% of the planned dose measured at the dorsum of the right foot was correlated with neuropathic pain intensities. Change of −0.05 °C in CDT had a sensitivity and specificity of 92.3% (95% CI 64.0% to 99.8%) 64.9% (95% CI 47.5% to 79.8%), respectively, in predicting neuropathic pain six months after finishing OXAIPN. For change in HPT and the prediction of neuropathic pain, −0.85 °C had a sensitivity of 64.3% (95% CI 35.1–87.2%) and a specificity of 70.0% (95% CI 53.5–83.4%) [59]. Conversely, no association in cold and warm thresholds in 35 cancer patients treated with OXA-based regimen and OXAIPN was identified [82].

The role of QST to early identify OXAIPN remains vaguely defined. Among limitations, technically challenging methods of QST are not widely available, are time-consuming, and need standardized assessment algorithms and normative data which are not universally defined [83,84]. Besides, QST requires patient's collaboration because results are based on a subjective response of the patient, compromising the objectivity desirable in a biomarker, and make QST not applicable in a subset of patients with impaired cognition and attention. Among QST parameters, VPT has the advantage of being quickly performed. Additionally, the equipment required is very portable and requires only basic training to operate. Accordingly, our and other authors experience [69] would favor VDT as the simplest and best routine marker among QST for detecting early OXAIPN in the clinic setting.

Other devices to quantify tactile sensation (Bumps Detection test) [42,81] or small fiber (Sudoscan) [85] have been investigated for early diagnosis of large or small fiber impairments in subjects suspected of having OXAIPN, and for monitoring change over time, with promising albeit very preliminary results. Baseline deficits in sensory functioning measured using the Bumps Detection test were predictive of increasing numbness/tingling during the first 26 weeks of OXA-based chemotherapy [81]. Very recently, a multicenter study including 101 patients evaluated the usefulness of the CLIP test for early prediction of the risk of progression ≥grade 2 neuropathy in patients receiving chemotherapy with OXA. By testing the difficulty of patients in picking up and moving five gem clips one by one two squares and assessing patients experience in performing the test, authors identified that a positive result on the CLIP test (by asking patient to pick up and move a gem clip and whether there was some wrongness in doing it) was associated with an 8.3-fold higher risk of progression to ≥grade 2 OXAIPN. Noteworthy, a positive conversion of the CLIP test occurred before the progression to ≥grade 2 OXAIPN in 14 of the 21 (67%) patients [86]. The usefulness of this simple, cheap, and widely available assessment tool should be further validated in larger, multicenter prospective comparative studies.

3.3. Axonal Excitability and Skin Biopsy

OXA produces acute changes in peripheral nerve excitability by modulating axonal voltage-gated Na^+ channel activity [74,87]. Nerve excitability studies evaluate axonal excitability to provide information of the properties of the nerve membrane and of the ion channels expressed on these axons [88]. Acute symptoms after OXA infusion correlate with nerve excitability findings [56]. This method can assess acute OXA-induced abnormalities in sensory or motor nerve function [56], and its cold-triggered aggravation [89].

Measurement of excitability parameters have been consistently shown to be a sensitive early biomarker of ongoing OXAIPN, even preceding the reduction in the SNAP and development of symptoms [76,90,91]. Patients who demonstrated changes in excitability in early treatment, shortly after infusion, were subsequently more likely to develop moderate to severe neurotoxicity. Park et al. reported that an increase in the superexcitability of more than 15% prior to 5 of 12 chemotherapy cycles was able to identify 80% of patients with moderate or severe chronic OXAIPN. Acute changes in axonal excitability parameters that developed in early treatment cycles anticipated development of later neurotoxicity in patients who completed seven or more treatment cycles. Patients who completed treatment with moderate to severe neurotoxicity showed greater changes in early treatment (cycles 1 or 2), particularly reductions in the associated hyperexcitability [76]. Despite OXA causes acute excitability changes in both motor and sensory axons, progressive cumulative changes were only found in sensory nerves, and motor nerve excitability studies did not reveal early cumulative changes following treatment with OXA [69,76].

Nerve excitability testing provides a sodium channel dysfunction index and an objective biomarker of acute OXA neurotoxicity useful to improve prediction and risk stratification for OXAIPN prior to the onset of chronic neuropathy [56]. However, their scarce availability in most of centers, time-consuming nature and the lack of standardization for the clinical testing [88], converts this technique in too complex for routine screening, and not applicable in daily clinical practice for early detection of OXAIPN.

Skin biopsy is a minimally invasive method to evaluate neuropathy, especially small fiber nerve damage. Five prospective studies have incorporated skin biopsy in assessing ongoing OXAIPN. Contradictory results on the change over time of intraepidermal nerve fiber (IEFN) are available [59,60,64,92,93]. No significant early reduction in IENF during OXA treatment has been demonstrated; evidence which could be related with the fact that loss of IENF, a marker of axonal degeneration, is usually a later event occurring in peripheral nerves [60,84]. Besides, ongoing regeneration of small nerve fibers during OXA could contribute to these discrepancies [59]. Therefore, skin biopsy should not be used for predicting OXAIPN.

4. Pharmacogenomic Biomarkers

Genetic factors may contribute to a patient's risk of experiencing OXAIPN. Over the last years, the development of pharmacogenetics, used to characterize human genetic variation, facilitated extensive efforts to understand the genetic basis of OXAIPN and to identify a specific genetic profile that can identify patients who are more liable to severe chronic neurotoxicity at the end of treatment. The majority of published studies assessed individual OXAIPN susceptibilities on single nucleotide polymorphisms (SNPs), which are mainly associated with gene variations in detoxification enzymes; DNA repair; drug transport; metabolism; neuronal receptors and ion channels (Figure 3). Furthermore, other genome wide analysis studies (GWAS) attempted to identify and validate SNPs mainly in genes encoding proteins implicated to neuronal function [94,95].

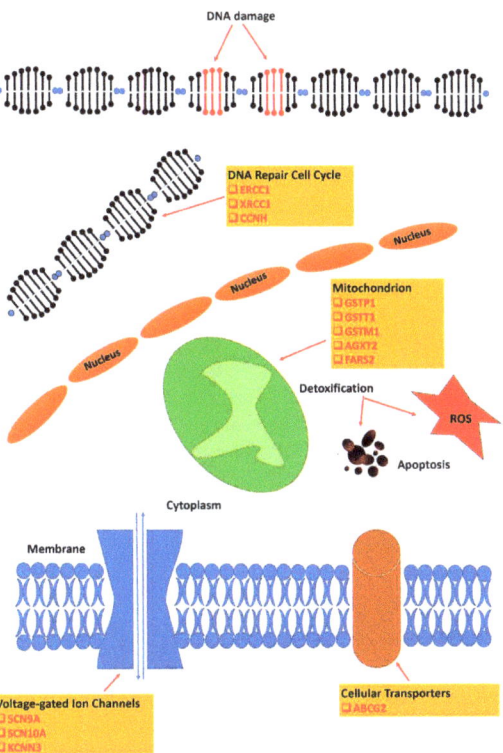

Figure 3. Cellular processes and main candidate genes implicated in oxaliplatin-induced neurotoxicity.

Some of these studies are of interest; tellingly, however, they have provided inconsistent findings and failed, in principle, to be replicated by other independent groups because of significant methodological limitations, including small sample sizes; retrospective study design; implementation of a post hoc analysis of oncology-based databases of different, not pre-planned size; lack of a pre-study hypothesis based on the known role of the investigated targets in the peripheral nervous system; inappropriate outcome measures for neurological impairment and differences related to DNA origin, extraction and genotyping [96].

4.1. SNP Studies

4.1.1. Glutathione-S-Transferase P1 (GSTP1), Glutathione-S-Transferase T1 (GSTT1) and Glutathione-S-Transferase M1 (GSTM1) Genotyping

Genetic variants for GSTP1 exon 5 (Ile105Val), GSTP1 exon 6 (Ala114Val), GSTM1 (homozygous deletion), and GSTT1 (homozygous deletion) were examined in a cohort of 64 OXA-treated CRC patients, among whom 15 had grade 3 chronic OXAIPN. Patients homozygous for the GSTP1 105Ile allele more frequently encountered grade 3 OXAIPN compared to patients homozygous or heterozygous for the GSTP1 105Val allele (OR: 5.75; 95% CI: 1.08–30.74; p = 0.02). GSTM1, GSTT1, or GSTP1 exon 6 genotypes have not been associated with severe chronic OXAIPN [97]. In another study enrolling 63 OXA-treated (mFOLFOX6) metastatic CRC patients, it was shown that GSTP1–105 (p = 0.03) and GSTM1 (p = 0.02) were associated with increased incidence of severe chronic OXAIPN [98]. Another two studies disclosed a significantly reduced risk of OXAIPN with the GSTP1 AA genotype (Ile/Ile) [99,100], while the same increased risk of OXAIPN manifestation was reported with the GG (Val/Val) genotype [101,102]. Noteworthy, there are several reports with controversial results showing no association of GSTP1 Ile105Val with increased incidence of OXAIPN [103–105].

4.1.2. ATP-Binding Cassette Transporter 2 (ABCG2) Genotyping

Custodio et al. performed genotyping in a cohort of 206 stage II-III OXA-treated CRC patients and a validation set of another 181 patients. Significant associations emerged for the CCNH rs2230641 C/C (OR: 5.03, 95% CI: 1.061–2.41, $p = 0.042$) and the ABCG2 rs3114018 A/A alleles (OR:2.67; 95% CI: 0.95–4.41; $p = 0.059$) with higher risk of grade 2–3 OXAIPN, while patients harboring the combination of these genotypes had significantly increased risk of severe OXAIPN, compared to patients carrying the CCNH any T and ABCG2 any C genotypes (37.73% vs. 19.42%; OR:2.46; 95% CI: 1.19–5.07; $p = 0.014$) [106].

However, replication of these results failed to achieve in a subsequent study enrolling 465 stage II or III CRC patients of Asian origin who were treated with the adjuvant-modified FOLFOX6 regimen. In the latter setting, comparison of low grade (0/1) OXAIPN with significant grade 2/3 OXAIPN did not showed any significant associations with any of the 12 examined SNP markers, including ABCG2 rs3114018 and CCNH rs2230641 [107]. In line with these negative results concerning the relevance of ABCG2 SNPs with OXAIPN, are the findings of a recently published study that tested germline DNA from 120 OXA-treated CRC patients together with a validation cohort of 80 patients and found no significant associations between ABCG2 (c.421 C > A/rs2231142) and increased incidence of OX-AIPN [108].

4.1.3. Cyclin-H (CCNH) Genotyping

The association of CCNH rs2230641 C/C with an increased incidence of severe OX-AIPN has been demonstrated in the Custodio et al.'s study (2014), which was mentioned earlier [106]. Furthermore, the same effect of CCNH genotypes in acute OXAIPN was demonstrated in another study enrolling 228 OXA-treated digestive tract cancer patients. This study revealed that the CCNH-rs2230641 (AA vs. AG+GG; dominant model) and CCNH-rs3093816 (AA vs. AG+GG; dominant model) were both found significant for higher risk of more frequent and severe acute OXAIPN [109].

4.1.4. X-ray Repair Cross-Complementing Protein 1 (XRCC) Genotyping

Genetic variants of the XRCC1 G/G polymorphism, which results in an Arg399Gln substitution has been tested for OXAIPN relevance in a study prospectively enrolling 292 Korean patients treated with FOLFOX for CRC and found that patients harboring XRCC1 23885GG experienced less grade 2–4 OXAIPN (adjusted OR:0.52, 95% CI: 0.27–0.99) [110].

Nonetheless, many other studies reported concordant evidence for lack of relevance between XRCC1 SNPs and OXAIPN, including Arg399Gln substitution [106,111]; Arg194Trp [112]; Arg280His [106,112]; rs3213239 [112]; rs12611088 and rs3213255 [106]. Subsequently published studies further provided evidence in support of the absence of any relevance of XRCC1 variants to OXAIPN features [105,107]. Tellingly, however, in the Kanai et al. study (2016), the proportions of patients developing grade 2–3 OXAIPN was quite higher compared to the Ruzzo et al.'s study (2014) (40.2% vs. 25.5).

4.1.5. Voltage-Gated Sodium Channels (SCNA) Genotyping

The SCN2A R19K polymorphism failed to be associated with liability to OXAIPN in a study in which 62 advanced CRC patients were genotyped [113]. Similarly, no significant association emerged between SCN9A variant rs6746030 and OXAIPN in a subsequent study comprising 200 CRC patients [114], contrasting the results of a smaller study in which SCN9A rs6746030 was protective of severe OXAIPN in a heterogeneous population of 94 patients with various digestive tract cancers, and an increased incidence of coexisting diabetes (24%) in patients with grade 3–4 OXAIPN [115]. Tellingly however, a subsequently published study performed genotyping in 228 Indian OXA-treated digestive tract cancer patients and found increased susceptibility to chronic OXAIPN with the rs6746030 polymorphic variant of SCN9A (GA+AA vs. GG: OR: 1.8; 95% CI:1.04–3.4; p = 0.04; dominant model), while the SCN10A polymorphic variant was associated with severity of chronic OXAIPN (OR:2.0; 95% CI:1.2–3.3; p = 0.006) [11].

Finally, in the Argyriou et al. study (2013), it was disclosed a significant association between the SCN4A variant rs2302237 and increased risk of any grade chronic OXAIPN (OR:2.47; 95% CI: 1.04–5.85; p = 0.037) and more severe acute OXAIPN (OR: 2.50; 95% CI:1.35–4.63; p = 0.0029) [114].

4.1.6. Voltage-Gated Potassium Channels (KCCN3) Genotyping

Basso et al. (2011) provided evidence for a significant association between 13–14 CAG repeat allele of KCNN3 (SK3) gene and development of acute OXAIPN (OR with >15 repeats; 0.381, 85% CI: 0.247–0.590, p = 0.001) in a small cohort of 40 CRC patients [116]. Another study, enrolling 86 CRC patients, did not show a significant association between chronic OXAIPN and KCNN3 repeat polymorphism [117]; concurring with the same negative results of a larger study studying 151 CRC patients and which provided evidence for lack of significant association between variations of the KCNN3 repeat polymorphism and development of either acute or chronic OXAIPN [113]. In any case, several mechanistic insights in OXAIPN pathogenesis are not supportive for a significant and direct involvement of K+channels in OXAIPN manifestation [118].

4.2. GWAS Studies

Won et al. (2012) performed GWAS in a discovery set of 96 and a validation cohort of 247 OXA-treated CRC patients of Asian origin in order to identify potential genetic markers for severe OXAIPN. This study identified and validated nine SNPs in eight genes [119], that failed to replicate in an independent validation in Caucasian patients [120]. The different genetic background of patients in the original and replication GWAS might hold the main response for conflicting results. No association was found with SNPs in ERCC1, GSTP1, XRCC1 and SNCA1 [119]. Finally, a very recently published study, enrolling over 1000 patients treated with paclitaxel, paclitaxel plus carboplatin, or oxaliplatin reported significant associations between rs56360211 near PDE6C (p = 7.92 × 10^{-8}) and rs113807868 near TMEM150C (p = 1.27 × 10^{-8}) with peripheral neurotoxicity. Tellingly, however, these results emerged from a polled analysis of treated patients and genetic associations were not tailored according to different chemotherapy compounds delivered [121].

There is increasing evidence pointing to the role of pharmacogenetics and pharmacogenomics in neurotoxicity susceptibility to OXA. Whereas pharmacogenetic results are currently being used in clinical decision making to inform treatment regimen choice with agents such as anthracycline [122] or fluoropyrimidine [123], larger-scale and validation studies are needed to further identify susceptibility markers of OXAIPN and to develop pharmacogenomics based-risk profiling to improve quality of life of gastrointestinal cancer patients.

5. Imaging Biomarkers

Data on imaging biomarkers in OXA-treated patients are still very limited, despite the benefit of their non-invasive nature. Nerve size, estimated by cross-sectional area (CSA), measured by nerve high-resolution ultrasound (HRUS), is an imaging modality that allows a quantitative structural analysis of the nerves. Existing clinical data on the application of HRUS in early assessment of OXAIPN are restricted to two small-sample-size studies. In 2013, Briani et al. conducted a cross-sectional study exploring the use of nerve HRUS in a cohort of 15 oxaliplatin-treated patients. The results showed an increased in CSA at common entrapment sites in 9 out of 15 patients prior to clinical symptoms and neurophysiological changes. At the end, 13 of the 15 patients developed a sensory axonal neuropathy [124]. More recently, Pitarokoili et al. conducted a prospective study on 13 oxaliplatin treated patients confirming an increase in CSA at upper limb entrapment sites and figuring out a CSA enlargement in tibial and fibular nerves. These findings also appeared either prior to or simultaneously with clinical and neurophysiology OXAIPN detection. No correlation between nerve HRUS, clinical severity and neurophysiology abnormalities was detected [125]. Moreover, a cross-sectional study of magnetic resonance neurography (MRN) in OXAIPN reported a significant dorsal root ganglia (DRG) hypertrophy after evaluating 20 patients. This finding correlates with one of the major mechanisms described for the initiation of neurotoxicity induced by this agent: the accumulation of platinum-DNA adducts in DRG [3]. Further investigation is required to establish the role of MRN as predictor of OXAIPN. Corneal confocal microscopy (CCM) is an ophthalmic noninvasive imaging modality that provides information of small sensory fibers by direct observation and scanning of corneal innervation with high resolution and magnification. Two prospective studies in gastrointestinal cancer patients are available, with conflicting results. Campagnolo M et al. demonstrated a reduction in the number and density of the corneal fibers after chemotherapy completion in 15 oxaliplatin treated patients [126]. Conversely, another study using CCM in 13 patients with upper GI cancer, eight of them who received 3 cycles of OXA containing regimes, identified a significant increase in corneal nerve fibre length [127].

Besides neuroimaging, other imaging techniques have been explored as surrogate biomarkers of early neurotoxicity. Preliminary evidences of the analysis body composition by computed tomography (CT) in gastrointestinal cancer patients reveal the loss of lean body muscle [128] or sarcopenic obesity [29] were independently associated with the occurrence of OXAIPN, supporting its potential predictive usefulness that deserves further investigation. Other radiologic measures including spleen volumetric analysis in CT scan [129] or muscle ultrasound [130] have been anecdotically explored in OXAIPN. To date, further larger research in imaging techniques is needed to provide further in-depth objective evidence in order to transfer them into daily clinical practice as predictive biomarkers of OXAIPN.

6. Blood Biomarkers

Several whole blood biomarkers have been investigated as predictive tools in the assessment of OXAIPN. Neurofilament light chain (NfL) is a neuron-specific cytoskeletal protein expressed in large-myelinated axons [131] released in blood when nerve damage occurs. Supported by a preclinical studies in vincristine-induced peripheral neuropathy [132], Kim et al. conducted a prospective study including 43 patients treated with OXA and measured serum NfLs during (at 3 months) and post-treatment (at 6 months). An increase in NfL levels in both periods was observed, being higher at 6 months of OXA-treatment. High serum NfL levels correlated with neuropathy severity, providing compelling evidence of NfLs as a potential predictive marker of OXAIPN. Interestingly, after 4–6 months of follow-up a meaningful reduction on NfL levels was observed, indicating that NfLs can also discriminate recovery patients from OXAIPN [133]. Despite promising, the predictive usefulness of NfL as a biomarker requires independent validation with further studies with larger sample sizes that allow researchers to establish universal reference values in order to maximize the correct interpretation of NfL in the management of OXAIPN [131].

Preclinical evidences showed a significant reduction in Nerve Growth Factor (NGF) levels during OXA administration in rat [134], which was correlated with the onset of peripheral neuropathy. Considering clinical studies, limited data is available. Velasco et al. conducted a prospective observational study including 60 cancer patients, of which 35 were OXA-treated with. The objective was to investigate the changes in circulating NGF levels and IENF in the presence or absence of neuropathic pain [93]. This research was based on the rationale that NGF receptor, TrKA, is located in the terminals of sensory neurons. Thus, the interaction between NGF and its receptor activates intracellular pathways affecting the sensitivity of nociceptors. The results of the study demonstrated an association between increased NGF levels and patients developing painful chemotherapy-induced peripheral neuropathy (CIPN), whereas NGF levels remained stable in patients with either painless or absent CIPN. Additionally, NGF level increases correlated with the severity of neuropathic pain reported by patients. However, no association between NGF levels and IENF was detected. Despite these promising results, previous studies did not report this association, therefore the role of NGF as a biomarker for the severity of painful OXAIPN remains unclear.

Other parameters routinely available from whole blood have been reported potentially useful in predicting the development of OXAIPN (Table 1). Pretreatment low hemoglobin level or anemia has been identified as a risk prognostic factor for OXAIPN in several studies. Mizrahi et al. carried out a large cross-sectional study including 105 patients treated with OXA. The results showed a correlation between reduced pretreatment levels of hemoglobin, detected in 24.5% of the cohort, with a greater severity of neuropathy [14]. In addition, previous studies on patients receiving OXA concluded similar results [15,19,22,27]. At pathophysiological level, a plausible explanation relating low hemoglobin levels and chronic neurotoxicity development is still unknown.

Among pretreatment metabolic and nutritional blood-based biomarkers, there are conflicting results. Such as higher albumin level [14] as hypoalbuminemia [15,19] have been associated with the risk of developing OXAIPN. Despite higher rates of neurotoxicity were described in patients with low levels of magnesium, the lack of evidence in this line [14] would support the known inefficacy of calcium-magnesium supplementation during OXA treatment as a neuroprotective approach [9]. Very recently and for the first time, higher serum gamma-glutamyl transferase (GGT) and a lower level of vitamin D have been identified as independent predictors of grade 2–3 OXAIPN in the multivariate analysis of a retrospective study including 186 gastrointestinal cancer patients [19]. Despite their easy collection and measure, non-invasiveness and objective interpretation of the results make blood tests perfect candidates to monitor neurotoxicity, more research is needed to better understand the pathophysiologic mechanisms underlying its role as prognostic biomarkers.

7. Conclusions

Early detection of OXAIPN is essential in the prevention of irreversible nerve damage and should be prioritized when assessing and evaluating patients receiving OXA treatment so that adequate adjustment in scheduled treatment plan can be made. Early clinical and neurophysiological signs of OXAIPN can be observed after low doses of OXA. The assessment of acute neurotoxicity symptoms in the routine clinical evaluation is a reliable biomarker for predicting the occurrence and development of OXAIPN, and particularly, the first cycles can be very informative. Regarding neurological examination, conflicting evidence on the timing of the threshold impairments hamper their currently use to inform clinicians in the prophylaxis of neuropathy. The development of a clinical standardized prognostic neuropathy assessment tool in order to early detect neuropathy should be validated. Despite, currently not part of common oncology practice, neurological monitoring with NCS may provide valuable reliable metric data in accurately disclosing and following the course of OXAIPN over time, offering at the same time useful information for dose reduction or discontinuation of the treatment before the progression to severe OXAIPN. Additionally, screening methods incorporating pharmacogenetics, may help to predict OXAIPN on the basis of genetic susceptibility and, consequently, allow a better, more personalized treatment. The further identification and validation of the simplest, non-invasive reliable and valid blood biomarkers for the premature screening of OXAIPN to reduce the morbidity and impairment in the quality of life of patients with gastrointestinal cancers associated with chronic OXAIPN might be of particular interest in neuroprotection trials. In the next future, by combining clinical, neurophysiological, genetic and potentially serum-based risks, decision-making would be improved to optimize treatment and prevent potentially serious neurotoxicity. The best noninvasive and easy-to-perform objective method to early detect and follow OXAIPN progression in the daily clinical practice in the hospital setting warrants further investigation and validation in larger prospective studies.

Author Contributions: Conceptualization, R.V. and A.A.A.; methodology, R.V., M.A., M.V. and A.A.A. writing—original draft preparation, R.V., M.A., M.V. and A.A.A.; writing—review and editing, R.V. and A.A.A.; supervision, R.V.; project administration, R.V.; funding acquisition, R.V. All authors have read and agreed to the published version of the manuscript.

Funding: This work was partially supported by a grant from Instituto de Salud Carlos III through the project PI20/00283 (Co-funded by European Regional Development Fund (ERDF)). We also thank CERCA Programme/Generalitat de Catalunya for institutional support.

Institutional Review Board Statement: Not applicable.

Informed Consent Statement: Not applicable.

Data Availability Statement: Data sharing not applicable.

Conflicts of Interest: The authors declare no conflict of interest. The funders had no role in the design of the study; in the collection, analyses, or interpretation of data; in the writing of the manuscript, or in the decision to publish the results.

Abbreviations

ABCG2	ATP-binding cassette transporter 2
AGXT2	Alanine-Glyoxylate Aminotransferase 2
CCNH	Cyclin-H
CCM	Corneal confocal microscopy
CIPN	Chemotherapy-Induced Peripheral Neuropathy
CRC	Colorectal Cancer
CMAP	Motor action compound potential
CSA	Cross-sectional area
CT	Computed Tomography
DRG	Dorsal root ganglia
ERCC1	Excision Repair 1, Endonuclease Non-Catalytic Subunit
FARS:2	Phenylalanyl-tRNA synthase 2
FOLFOX	Folinic acid, 5-fluorouracil, and oxaliplatin
FOLFIRINOX	Fluorouracil leucovorin irinotecan oxaliplatin
GSTP1	Glutathione-S-transferase P1
GSTM1	Glutathione-S-transferase M1
GSTT1	Glutathione-S-transferase T1
GWAS	Genome wide analysis studies
HRUS	High-resolution ultrasound
IENF	Intraepidermal nerve fiber
KCCN3	Voltage-gated potassium channels
MRN	Magnetic resonance neurography
NCI-CTCAE	Common Terminology Criteria for Adverse Events from the National Cancer Institute
NCS	Nerve Conduction Studies
NGF	Nerve Growth Factor
NfL	Neurofilament light chain
OXA	Oxaliplatin
OXAIPN	Oxaliplatin-induced peripheral neurotoxicity
QST	Quantitative Sensory Testing
ROS	Reactive oxygen species
SCNA	Voltage-gated sodium channels
SNP	Single nucleotide polymorphism
SNAP	Sensory nerve action potential
XELOX	capecitabine and oxaliplatin
XRCC:1	X-ray repair cross-complementing protein 1

References

1. Conroy, T.; Hammel, P.; Hebbar, M.; Ben Abdelghani, M.; Wei, A.C.; Raoul, J.-L.; Choné, L.; Francois, E.; Artru, P.; Biagi, J.J.; et al. FOLFIRINOX or Gemcitabine as Adjuvant Therapy for Pancreatic Cancer. *N. Engl. J. Med.* **2018**, *379*, 2395–2406. [CrossRef] [PubMed]
2. André, T.; Boni, C.; Navarro, M.; Tabernero, J.; Hickish, T.; Topham, C.; Bonetti, A.; Clingan, P.; Bridgewater, J.; Rivera, F.; et al. Improved Overall Survival with Oxaliplatin, Fluorouracil, and Leucovorin As Adjuvant Treatment in Stage II or III Colon Cancer in the MOSAIC Trial. *JCO* **2009**, *27*, 3109–3116. [CrossRef]
3. Velasco, R.; Bruna, J. Oxaliplatin Neurotoxicity. *Curr. Colorectal Cancer Rep.* **2014**, *10*, 303–312. [CrossRef]
4. Yamaguchi, K.; Kusaba, H.; Makiyama, A.; Mitsugi, K.; Uchino, K.; Tamura, S.; Shibata, Y.; Esaki, T.; Ito, M.; Takayoshi, K.; et al. The risk factors for oxaliplatin-induced peripheral sensory neuropathy and thrombocytopenia in advanced gastric cancer. *Cancer Chemother. Pharm.* **2018**, *82*, 625–633. [CrossRef] [PubMed]
5. Beijers, A.J.M.; Mols, F.; Tjan-Heijnen, V.C.G.; Faber, C.G.; van de Poll-Franse, L.V.; Vreugdenhil, G. Peripheral neuropathy in colorectal cancer survivors: The influence of oxaliplatin administration. Results from the population-based PROFILES registry. *Acta Oncol.* **2015**, *54*, 463–469. [CrossRef]
6. Besora, S.; Santos, C.; Izquierdo, C.; Martinez-Villacampa, M.M.; Bruna, J.; Velasco, R. Rechallenge with oxaliplatin and peripheral neuropathy in colorectal cancer patients. *J. Cancer Res. Clin. Oncol.* **2018**, *144*, 1793–1801. [CrossRef]
7. Argyriou, A.A.; Kalofonou, F.; Litsardopoulos, P.; Anastopoulou, G.G.; Kalofonos, H.P. Oxaliplatin rechallenge in metastatic colorectal cancer patients with clinically significant oxaliplatin-induced peripheral neurotoxicity. *J. Peripher. Nerv. Syst.* **2021**, *26*, 43–48. [CrossRef]
8. Selvy, M.; Pereira, B.; Kerckhove, N.; Gonneau, C.; Feydel, G.; Pétorin, C.; Vimal-Baguet, A.; Melnikov, S.; Kullab, S.; Hebbar, M.; et al. Long-Term Prevalence of Sensory Chemotherapy-Induced Peripheral Neuropathy for 5 Years after Adjuvant FOLFOX Chemotherapy to Treat Colorectal Cancer: A Multicenter Cross-Sectional Study. *JCM* **2020**, *9*, 2400. [CrossRef] [PubMed]
9. Loprinzi, C.L.; Lacchetti, C.; Bleeker, J.; Cavaletti, G.; Chauhan, C.; Hertz, D.L.; Kelley, M.R.; Lavino, A.; Lustberg, M.B.; Paice, J.A.; et al. Prevention and Management of Chemotherapy-Induced Peripheral Neuropathy in Survivors of Adult Cancers: ASCO Guideline Update. *JCO* **2020**, *38*, 3325–3348. [CrossRef] [PubMed]
10. Gebremedhn, E.G.; Shortland, P.J.; Mahns, D.A. The incidence of acute oxaliplatin-induced neuropathy and its impact on treatment in the first cycle: A systematic review. *BMC Cancer* **2018**, *18*, 410. [CrossRef]
11. Palugulla, S.; Dkhar, S.; Kayal, S.; Narayan, S. Oxaliplatin-induced peripheral neuropathy in south indian cancer patients: A prospective study in digestive tract cancer patients. *Indian J. Med. Paediatr Oncol.* **2017**, *38*, 502. [CrossRef]
12. Alejandro, L.M.; Behrendt, C.E.; Chen, K.; Openshaw, H.; Shibata, S. Predicting Acute and Persistent Neuropathy Associated With Oxaliplatin. *Am. J. Clin. Oncol.* **2013**, *36*, 331–337. [CrossRef]
13. Hsu, S.; Huang, W.; Lee, S.; Chu, T.; Lin, Y.; Lu, C.; Beaton, R.D.; Jane, S. Incidence, severity, longitudinal trends and predictors of acute and chronic oxaliplatin-induced peripheral neuropathy in Taiwanese patients with colorectal cancer. *Eur. J. Cancer Care* **2018**, e12976. [CrossRef]
14. Mizrahi, D.; Park, S.B.; Li, T.; Timmins, H.C.; Trinh, T.; Au, K.; Battaglini, E.; Wyld, D.; Henderson, R.D.; Grimison, P.; et al. Hemoglobin, Body Mass Index, and Age as Risk Factors for Paclitaxel- and Oxaliplatin-Induced Peripheral Neuropathy. *JAMA Netw. Open* **2021**, *4*, e2036695. [CrossRef] [PubMed]
15. Vincenzi, B.; Frezza, A.M.; Schiavon, G.; Spoto, C.; Addeo, R.; Catalano, V.; Graziano, F.; Santini, D.; Tonini, G. Identification of clinical predictive factors of oxaliplatin-induced chronic peripheral neuropathy in colorectal cancer patients treated with adjuvant Folfox IV. *Support. Care Cancer* **2013**, *21*, 1313–1319. [CrossRef]
16. Raphael, M.J.; Fischer, H.D.; Fung, K.; Austin, P.C.; Anderson, G.M.; Booth, C.M.; Singh, S. Neurotoxicity Outcomes in a Population-based Cohort of Elderly Patients Treated With Adjuvant Oxaliplatin for Colorectal Cancer. *Clin. Colorectal Cancer* **2017**, *16*, 397–404.e1. [CrossRef]
17. Velasco, R.; Bruna, J.; Briani, C.; Argyriou, A.A.; Cavaletti, G.; Alberti, P.; Frigeni, B.; Cacciavillani, M.; Lonardi, S.; Cortinovis, D.; et al. Early predictors of oxaliplatin-induced cumulative neuropathy in colorectal cancer patients. *J. Neurol. Neurosurg. Psychiatry* **2014**, *85*, 392–398. [CrossRef] [PubMed]
18. Pulvers, J.N.; Marx, G. Factors associated with the development and severity of oxaliplatin-induced peripheral neuropathy: A systematic review. *Asia-Pac. J. Clin. Oncol.* **2017**, *13*, 345–355. [CrossRef] [PubMed]
19. Yildirim, N.; Cengiz, M. Predictive clinical factors of chronic peripheral neuropathy induced by oxaliplatin. *Support. Care Cancer* **2020**, *28*, 4781–4788. [CrossRef] [PubMed]
20. Attal, N.; Bouhassira, D.; Gautron, M.; Vaillant, J.N.; Mitry, E.; Lepère, C.; Rougier, P.; Guirimand, F. Thermal hyperalgesia as a marker of oxaliplatin neurotoxicity: A prospective quantified sensory assessment study. *Pain* **2009**, *144*, 245–252. [CrossRef]
21. Argyriou, A.A.; Briani, C.; Cavaletti, G.; Bruna, J.; Alberti, P.; Velasco, R.; Lonardi, S.; Cortinovis, D.; Cazzaniga, M.; Campagnolo, M.; et al. Advanced age and liability to oxaliplatin-induced peripheral neuropathy: Post hoc analysis of a prospective study. *Eur. J. Neurol.* **2013**, *20*, 788–794. [CrossRef]
22. Sugihara, K.; Ohtsu, A.; Shimada, Y.; Mizunuma, N.; Gomi, K.; Lee, P.; Gramont, A.; Rothenberg, M.L.; André, T.; Brienza, S.; et al. Analysis of neurosensory adverse events induced by FOLFOX 4 treatment in colorectal cancer patients: A comparison between two Asian studies and four Western studies. *Cancer Med.* **2012**, *1*, 198–206. [CrossRef]

23. Baek, K.K.; Lee, J.; Park, S.H.; Park, J.O.; Park, Y.S.; Lim, H.Y.; Kang, W.K.; Cho, Y.B.; Yun, S.H.; Kim, H.C.; et al. Oxaliplatin-Induced Chronic Peripheral Neurotoxicity: A Prospective Analysis in Patients with Colorectal Cancer. *Cancer Res. Treat.* **2010**, *42*, 185. [CrossRef]
24. Wiela-Hojeńska, A.; Kowalska, T.; Filipczyk-Cisarż, E.; Łapiński, Ł.; Nartowski, K. Evaluation of the Toxicity of Anti-cancerChemotherapy in Patients with Colon Cancer. *Adv. Clin. Exp. Med.* **2015**, *24*, 103–111. [CrossRef]
25. Kim, J.; Ji, E.; Jung, K.; Jung, I.H.; Park, J.; Lee, J.-C.; Kim, J.W.; Hwang, J.-H.; Kim, J. Gender Differences in Patients with Metastatic Pancreatic Cancer Who Received FOLFIRINOX. *JPM* **2021**, *11*, 83. [CrossRef]
26. Nagata, T.; Fukuda, K.-I.; Tamai, M.; Taniguchi, A.; Kamiya, H.; Kambe, K.; Kamada, Y.; Iwata, G.; Yamaoka, N. Early Neuropathy Related to Oxaliplatin Treatment in Advanced and Recurrent Colorectal Cancer. *Anticancer Res.* **2019**, *39*, 1347–1353. [CrossRef] [PubMed]
27. Shahriari-Ahmadi, A.; Fahimi, A.; Payandeh, M.; Sadeghi, M. Prevalence of Oxaliplatin-induced Chronic Neuropathy and Influencing Factors in Patients with Colorectal Cancer in Iran. *Asian Pac. J. Cancer Prev.* **2015**, *16*, 7603–7606. [CrossRef] [PubMed]
28. Ottaiano, A.; Nappi, A.; Tafuto, S.; Nasti, G.; De Divitiis, C.; Romano, C.; Cassata, A.; Casaretti, R.; Silvestro, L.; Avallone, A.; et al. Diabetes and Body Mass Index Are Associated with Neuropathy and Prognosis in Colon Cancer Patients Treated with Capecitabine and Oxaliplatin Adjuvant Chemotherapy. *Oncology* **2016**, *90*, 36–42. [CrossRef]
29. Dijksterhuis, W.P.M.; Pruijt, M.J.; Woude, S.O.; Klaassen, R.; Kurk, S.A.; Oijen, M.G.H.; Laarhoven, H.W.M. Association between body composition, survival, and toxicity in advanced esophagogastric cancer patients receiving palliative chemotherapy. *J. Cachexia Sarcopenia Muscle* **2019**, *10*, 199–206. [CrossRef] [PubMed]
30. Kanbayashi, Y.; Hosokawa, T.; Okamoto, K.; Konishi, H.; Otsuji, E.; Yoshikawa, T.; Takagi, T.; Taniwaki, M. Statistical identification of predictors for peripheral neuropathy associated with administration of bortezomib, taxanes, oxaliplatin or vincristine using ordered logistic regression analysis. *Anti-Cancer Drugs* **2010**, *21*, 877–881. [CrossRef] [PubMed]
31. Giantonio, B.J.; Catalano, P.J.; Meropol, N.J.; O'Dwyer, P.J.; Mitchell, E.P.; Alberts, S.R.; Schwartz, M.A.; Benson, A.B. Bevacizumab in Combination With Oxaliplatin, Fluorouracil, and Leucovorin (FOLFOX4) for Previously Treated Metastatic Colorectal Cancer: Results From the Eastern Cooperative Oncology Group Study E3200. *JCO* **2007**, *25*, 1539–1544. [CrossRef]
32. Hochster, H.S.; Hart, L.L.; Ramanathan, R.K.; Childs, B.H.; Hainsworth, J.D.; Cohn, A.L.; Wong, L.; Fehrenbacher, L.; Abubakr, Y.; Saif, M.W.; et al. Safety and Efficacy of Oxaliplatin and Fluoropyrimidine Regimens With or Without Bevacizumab As First-Line Treatment of Metastatic Colorectal Cancer: Results of the TREE Study. *JCO* **2008**, *26*, 3523–3529. [CrossRef]
33. Hsu, T.-W.; Chen, F.-A.; Yao, Y.-H.; Wang, W.-S. Creatinine Clearance Rate and Nerve Conduction Velocity are Effective in Objectively Assessing Oxaliplatin-Neuropathy in Patients with Colorectal Carcinoma. *HGE* **2011**. [CrossRef]
34. Takimoto, C.H.; Graham, M.A.; Lockwood, G.; Ng, C.M.; Goetz, A.; Greenslade, D.; Remick, S.C.; Sharma, S.; Mani, S.; Ramanathan, R.K.; et al. Oxaliplatin Pharmacokinetics and Pharmacodynamics in Adult Cancer Patients with Impaired Renal Function. *Clin. Cancer Res.* **2007**, *13*, 4832–4839. [CrossRef] [PubMed]
35. Massari, C.; Brienza, S.; Rotarski, M.; Gastiaburu, J.; Misset, J.-L.; Cupissol, D.; Alafaci, E.; Dutertre-Catella, H.; Bastian, G. Pharmacokinetics of oxaliplatin in patients with normal versus impaired renal function. *Cancer Chemother. Pharm.* **2000**, *45*, 157–164. [CrossRef]
36. Watanabe, D.; Fujii, H.; Matsuhashi, N.; Iihara, H.; Yamada, Y.; Ishihara, T.; Takahashi, T.; Yoshida, K.; Suzuki, A. Dose Adjustment of Oxaliplatin Based on Renal Function in Patients With Metastatic Colorectal Cancer. *Anticancer Res.* **2020**, *40*, 2379–2386. [CrossRef] [PubMed]
37. Uwah, A.N.; Ackler, J.; Leighton, J.C.; Pomerantz, S.; Tester, W. The Effect of Diabetes on Oxaliplatin-Induced Peripheral Neuropathy. *Clin. Colorectal Cancer* **2012**, *11*, 275–279. [CrossRef] [PubMed]
38. Abdel-Rahman, O. Impact of diabetes comorbidity on the efficacy and safety of FOLFOX first-line chemotherapy among patients with metastatic colorectal cancer: A pooled analysis of two phase-III studies. *Clin. Transl. Oncol.* **2019**, *21*, 512–518. [CrossRef]
39. Ramanathan, R.K.; Rothenberg, M.L.; de Gramont, A.; Tournigand, C.; Goldberg, R.M.; Gupta, S.; André, T. Incidence and evolution of oxaliplatin-induced peripheral sensory neuropathy in diabetic patients with colorectal cancer: A pooled analysis of three phase III studies. *Ann. Oncol.* **2010**, *21*, 754–758. [CrossRef] [PubMed]
40. Wesselink, E.; Winkels, R.; van Baar, H.; Geijsen, A.; van Zutphen, M.; van Halteren, H.; Hansson, B.; Radema, S.; de Wilt, J.; Kampman, E.; et al. Dietary Intake of Magnesium or Calcium and Chemotherapy-Induced Peripheral Neuropathy in Colorectal Cancer Patients. *Nutrients* **2018**, *10*, 398. [CrossRef]
41. Banach, M.; Zygulska, A.; Krzemieniecki, K. Oxaliplatin treatment and peripheral nerve damage in cancer patients: A Polish cohort study. *J. Can. Res.* **2018**, *14*, 1010. [CrossRef]
42. de Carvalho Barbosa, M.; Kosturakis, A.K.; Eng, C.; Wendelschafer-Crabb, G.; Kennedy, W.R.; Simone, D.A.; Wang, X.S.; Cleeland, C.S.; Dougherty, P.M.A. Quantitative Sensory Analysis of Peripheral Neuropathy in Colorectal Cancer and Its Exacerbation by Oxaliplatin Chemotherapy. *Cancer Res.* **2014**, *74*, 5955–5962. [CrossRef]
43. Altaf, R.; Lund Brixen, A.; Kristensen, B.; Nielsen, S.E. Incidence of Cold-Induced Peripheral Neuropathy and Dose Modification of Adjuvant Oxaliplatin-Based Chemotherapy for Patients with Colorectal Cancer. *Oncology* **2014**, *87*, 167–172. [CrossRef] [PubMed]
44. Soveri, L.M.; Lamminmäki, A.; Hänninen, U.A.; Karhunen, M.; Bono, P.; Osterlund, P. Long-term neuropathy and quality of life in colorectal cancer patients treated with oxaliplatin containing adjuvant chemotherapy. *Acta Oncol.* **2019**, *58*, 398–406. [CrossRef] [PubMed]

45. Yoshino, T.; Yamanaka, T.; Oki, E.; Kotaka, M.; Manaka, D.; Eto, T.; Hasegawa, J.; Takagane, A.; Nakamura, M.; Kato, T.; et al. Efficacy and Long-term Peripheral Sensory Neuropathy of 3 vs 6 Months of Oxaliplatin-Based Adjuvant Chemotherapy for Colon Cancer: The ACHIEVE Phase 3 Randomized Clinical Trial. *JAMA Oncol.* **2019**, *5*, 1574. [CrossRef] [PubMed]
46. Argyriou, A.A.; Velasco, R.; Briani, C.; Cavaletti, G.; Bruna, J.; Alberti, P.; Cacciavillani, M.; Lonardi, S.; Santos, C.; Cortinovis, D.; et al. Peripheral neurotoxicity of oxaliplatin in combination with 5-fluorouracil (FOLFOX) or capecitabine (XELOX): A prospective evaluation of 150 colorectal cancer patients. *Ann. Oncol.* **2012**, *23*, 3116–3122. [CrossRef] [PubMed]
47. Iveson, T.J.; Sobrero, A.F.; Yoshino, T.; Souglakos, I.; Ou, F.-S.; Meyers, J.P.; Shi, Q.; Grothey, A.; Saunders, M.P.; Labianca, R.; et al. Duration of Adjuvant Doublet Chemotherapy (3 or 6 months) in Patients With High-Risk Stage II Colorectal Cancer. *JCO* **2021**, *39*, 631–641. [CrossRef]
48. Pachman, D.R.; Qin, R.; Seisler, D.K.; Smith, E.M.L.; Beutler, A.S.; Ta, L.E.; Lafky, J.M.; Wagner-Johnston, N.D.; Ruddy, K.J.; Dakhil, S.; et al. Clinical Course of Oxaliplatin-Induced Neuropathy: Results From the Randomized Phase III Trial N08CB (Alliance). *JCO* **2015**, *33*, 3416–3422. [CrossRef]
49. Tanishima, H.; Tominaga, T.; Kimura, M.; Maeda, T.; Shirai, Y.; Horiuchi, T. Hyperacute peripheral neuropathy is a predictor of oxaliplatin-induced persistent peripheral neuropathy. *Support. Care Cancer* **2017**, *25*, 1383–1389. [CrossRef]
50. Matsumoto, Y.; Yoshida, Y.; Kiba, S.; Yamashiro, S.; Nogami, H.; Ohashi, N.; Kajitani, R.; Munechika, T.; Nagano, H.; Komono, A.; et al. Acute chemotherapy-induced peripheral neuropathy due to oxaliplatin administration without cold stimulation. *Support. Care Cancer* **2020**, *28*, 5405–5410. [CrossRef]
51. Land, S.R.; Kopec, J.A.; Cecchini, R.S.; Ganz, P.A.; Wieand, H.S.; Colangelo, L.H.; Murphy, K.; Kuebler, J.P.; Seay, T.E.; Needles, B.M.; et al. Neurotoxicity From Oxaliplatin Combined With Weekly Bolus Fluorouracil and Leucovorin As Surgical Adjuvant Chemotherapy for Stage II and III Colon Cancer: NSABP C-07. *JCO* **2007**, *25*, 2205–2211. [CrossRef]
52. Argyriou, A.A.; Cavaletti, G.; Briani, C.; Velasco, R.; Bruna, J.; Campagnolo, M.; Alberti, P.; Bergamo, F.; Cortinovis, D.; Cazzaniga, M.; et al. Clinical pattern and associations of oxaliplatin acute neurotoxicity: A prospective study in 170 patients with colorectal cancer. *Cancer* **2013**, *119*, 438–444. [CrossRef]
53. Bruna, J.; Videla, S.; Argyriou, A.A.; Velasco, R.; Villoria, J.; Santos, C.; Nadal, C.; Cavaletti, G.; Alberti, P.; Briani, C.; et al. Efficacy of a Novel Sigma-1 Receptor Antagonist for Oxaliplatin-Induced Neuropathy: A Randomized, Double-Blind, Placebo-Controlled Phase IIa Clinical Trial. *Neurotherapeutics* **2018**, *15*, 178–189. [CrossRef]
54. Argyriou, A.A.; Kalofonou, F.; Litsardopoulos, P.; Anastopoulou, G.G.; Psimaras, D.; Bruna, J.; Kalofonos, H.P. Real world, open label experience with lacosamide against acute painful oxaliplatin-induced peripheral neurotoxicity. *J. Peripher. Nerv. Syst.* **2020**, *25*, 178–183. [CrossRef] [PubMed]
55. Van Den Heuvel, S.A.; Doorduin, J.; Steegers, M.A.H.; Bronkhorst, E.M.; Radema, S.A.; Vissers, K.C.P.; Van Der Wal, S.E.I.; Van Alfen, N. Simple surface EMG recording as a noninvasive screening method for the detection of acute oxaliplatin-induced neurotoxicity: A feasibility pilot study. *Neurosci. Lett.* **2019**, *699*, 184–188. [CrossRef] [PubMed]
56. Heide, R.; Bostock, H.; Ventzel, L.; Grafe, P.; Bergmans, J.; Fuglsang-Frederiksen, A.; Finnerup, N.B.; Tankisi, H. Axonal excitability changes and acute symptoms of oxaliplatin treatment: In vivo evidence for slowed sodium channel inactivation. *Clin. Neurophysiol.* **2018**, *129*, 694–706. [CrossRef]
57. Lucchetta, M.; Lonardi, S.; Bergamo, F.; Alberti, P.; Velasco, R.; Argyriou, A.A.; Briani, C.; Bruna, J.; Cazzaniga, M.; Cortinovis, D.; et al. Incidence of atypical acute nerve hyperexcitability symptoms in oxaliplatin-treated patients with colorectal cancer. *Cancer Chemother. Pharm.* **2012**, *70*, 899–902. [CrossRef]
58. Kokotis, P.; Schmelz, M.; Kostouros, E.; Karandreas, N.; Dimopoulos, M.-A. Oxaliplatin-Induced Neuropathy: A Long-Term Clinical and Neurophysiologic Follow-Up Study. *Clin. Colorectal Cancer* **2016**, *15*, e133–e140. [CrossRef]
59. Krøigård, T.; Svendsen, T.K.; Wirenfeldt, M.; Schrøder, H.D.; Qvortrup, C.; Pfeiffer, P.; Gaist, D.; Sindrup, S.H. Oxaliplatin neuropathy: Predictive values of skin biopsy, QST and nerve conduction. *JND* **2021**, 1–10. [CrossRef] [PubMed]
60. Krøigård, T.; Svendsen, T.K.; Wirenfeldt, M.; Schrøder, H.D.; Qvortrup, C.; Pfeiffer, P.; Gaist, D.; Sindrup, S.H. Early changes in tests of peripheral nerve function during oxaliplatin treatment and their correlation with chemotherapy-induced polyneuropathy symptoms and signs. *Eur. J. Neurol.* **2020**, *27*, 68–76. [CrossRef]
61. Pietrangeli, A.; Leandri, M.; Terzoli, E.; Jandolo, B.; Garufi, C. Persistence of High-Dose Oxaliplatin-Induced Neuropathy at Long-Term Follow-Up. *Eur. Neurol.* **2006**, *56*, 13–16. [CrossRef] [PubMed]
62. Argyriou, A.A.; Polychronopoulos, P.; Chroni, E. The Usefulness of Nerve Conduction Studies in Objectively Assessing Oxaliplatin-Induced Peripheral Neuropathy. *Oncologist* **2007**, *12*, 1371–1372. [CrossRef]
63. Kim, S.-H.; Kim, W.; Kim, J.-H.; Woo, M.K.; Baek, J.Y.; Kim, S.Y.; Chung, S.H.; Kim, H.J. A Prospective Study of Chronic Oxaliplatin-Induced Neuropathy in Patients with Colon Cancer: Long-Term Outcomes and Predictors of Severe Oxaliplatin-Induced Neuropathy. *J. Clin. Neurol.* **2018**, *14*, 81. [CrossRef] [PubMed]
64. Burakgazi, A.Z.; Messersmith, W.; Vaidya, D.; Hauer, P.; Hoke, A.; Polydefkis, M. Longitudinal assessment of oxaliplatin-induced neuropathy. *Neurology* **2011**, *77*, 980–986. [CrossRef] [PubMed]
65. de Gramont, A.; Figer, A.; Seymour, M.; Homerin, M.; Hmissi, A.; Cassidy, J.; Boni, C.; Cortes-Funes, H.; Cervantes, A.; Freyer, G.; et al. Leucovorin and Fluorouracil With or Without Oxaliplatin as First-Line Treatment in Advanced Colorectal Cancer. *JCO* **2000**, *18*, 2938–2947. [CrossRef] [PubMed]

66. Argyriou, A.A.; Bruna, J.; Anastopoulou, G.G.; Velasco, R.; Litsardopoulos, P.; Kalofonos, H.P. Assessing risk factors of falls in cancer patients with chemotherapy-induced peripheral neurotoxicity. *Support. Care Cancer* **2020**, *28*, 1991–1995. [CrossRef] [PubMed]
67. Takeshita, E.; Ishibashi, K.; Koda, K.; Oda, N.; Yoshimatsu, K.; Sato, Y.; Oya, M.; Yamaguchi, S.; Nakajima, H.; Momma, T.; et al. The updated five-year overall survival and long-term oxaliplatin-related neurotoxicity assessment of the FACOS study. *Surg. Today* **2021**. [CrossRef]
68. Yothers, G.; O'Connell, M.J.; Allegra, C.J.; Kuebler, J.P.; Colangelo, L.H.; Petrelli, N.J.; Wolmark, N. Oxaliplatin As Adjuvant Therapy for Colon Cancer: Updated Results of NSABP C-07 Trial, Including Survival and Subset Analyses. *JCO* **2011**, *29*, 3768–3774. [CrossRef]
69. Mc Hugh, J.C.; Tryfonopoulos, D.; Fennelly, D.; Crown, J.; Connolly, S. Electroclinical biomarkers of early peripheral neurotoxicity from oxaliplatin: Oxaliplatin neuropathy. *Eur. J. Cancer Care* **2012**, *21*, 782–789. [CrossRef]
70. Alberti, P.; Rossi, E.; Argyriou, A.A.; Kalofonos, H.P.; Briani, C.; Cacciavillani, M.; Campagnolo, M.; Bruna, J.; Velasco, R.; Cazzaniga, M.E.; et al. Risk stratification of oxaliplatin induced peripheral neurotoxicity applying electrophysiological testing of dorsal sural nerve. *Support. Care Cancer* **2018**, *26*, 3143–3151. [CrossRef]
71. Briani, C.; Argyriou, A.A.; Izquierdo, C.; Velasco, R.; Campagnolo, M.; Alberti, P.; Frigeni, B.; Cacciavillani, M.; Bergamo, F.; Cortinovis, D.; et al. Long-term course of oxaliplatin-induced polyneuropathy: A prospective 2-year follow-up study. *J. Peripher. Nerv. Syst.* **2014**, *19*, 299–306. [CrossRef]
72. Lehky, T.J.; Leonard, G.D.; Wilson, R.H.; Grem, J.L.; Floeter, M.K. Oxaliplatin-induced neurotoxicity: Acute hyperexcitability and chronic neuropathy. *Muscle Nerve* **2004**, *29*, 387–392. [CrossRef] [PubMed]
73. Wilson, R.H.; Lehky, T.; Thomas, R.R.; Quinn, M.G.; Floeter, M.K.; Grem, J.L. Acute Oxaliplatin-Induced Peripheral Nerve Hyperexcitability. *JCO* **2002**, *20*, 1767–1774. [CrossRef]
74. Hill, A.; Bergin, P.; Hanning, F.; Thompson, P.; Findlay, M.; Damianovich, D.; McKeage, M.J. Detecting acute neurotoxicity during platinum chemotherapy by neurophysiological assessment of motor nerve hyperexcitability. *BMC Cancer* **2010**, *10*, 451. [CrossRef] [PubMed]
75. Gebremedhn, E.G.; Shortland, P.J.; Mahns, D.A. Variability of Oxaliplatin-Induced Neuropathic Pain Symptoms in Each Cycle and Its Implications on the Management of Colorectal Cancer Patients: A Retrospective Study in South Western Sydney Local Health District Hospitals, Sydney, Australia. *J. Oncol.* **2019**, *2019*, 4828563. [CrossRef]
76. Park, S.B.; Lin, C.S.-Y.; Krishnan, A.V.; Goldstein, D.; Friedlander, M.L.; Kiernan, M.C. Oxaliplatin-induced neurotoxicity: Changes in axonal excitability precede development of neuropathy. *Brain* **2009**, *132*, 2712–2723. [CrossRef]
77. Forstenpointner, J.; Oberlojer, V.C.; Naleschinski, D.; Höper, J.; Helfert, S.M.; Andreas, B.; Gierthmühlen, J.; Ralf Baron, R. A-Fibers Mediate Cold Hyperalgesia in Patients with Oxaliplatin-Induced Neuropathy. *Pain Pract.* **2018**, *18*, 758–767. [CrossRef] [PubMed]
78. Godinho, P.A.R.; Silva, P.G.B.; Lisboa, M.R.P.; Costa, B.A.; Gifoni, M.A.C.; Rocha Filho, D.R.; Lima-Júnior, R.C.P.; Vale, M.L. Electronic von Frey as an objective assessment tool for oxaliplatin-induced peripheral neuropathy: A prospective longitudinal study. *Eur. J. Cancer Care* **2021**, *30*. [CrossRef]
79. Velasco, R.; Videla, S.; Villoria, J.; Ortiz, E.; Navarro, X.; Bruna, J. Reliability and accuracy of quantitative sensory testing for oxaliplatin-induced neurotoxicity. *Acta Neurol. Scand.* **2015**, *131*, 282–289. [CrossRef]
80. Reddy, S.M.; Vergo, M.T.; Paice, J.A.; Kwon, N.; Helenowski, I.B.; Benson, A.B.; Mulcahy, M.F.; Nimeiri, H.S.; Harden, R.N. Quantitative Sensory Testing at Baseline and During Cycle 1 Oxaliplatin Infusion Detects Subclinical Peripheral Neuropathy and Predicts Clinically Overt Chronic Neuropathy in Gastrointestinal Malignancies. *Clin. Colorectal Cancer* **2016**, *15*, 37–46. [CrossRef] [PubMed]
81. Wang, X.S.; Shi, Q.; Dougherty, P.M.; Eng, C.; Mendoza, T.R.; Williams, L.A.; Fogelman, D.R.; Cleeland, C.S. Prechemotherapy Touch Sensation Deficits Predict Oxaliplatin-Induced Neuropathy in Patients with Colorectal Cancer. *Oncology* **2016**, *90*, 127–135. [CrossRef]
82. Delmotte, J.; Beaussier, H.; Auzeil, N.; Massicot, F.; Laprévote, O.; Raymond, E.; Coudoré, F. Is quantitative sensory testing helpful in the management of oxaliplatin neuropathy? a two-year clinical study. *Cancer Treat. Res. Commun.* **2018**, *17*, 31–36. [CrossRef] [PubMed]
83. Williams, D.; Conn, J.; Talley, N.; Attia, J. Reviewing the evidence base for the peripheral sensory examination. *Int. J. Clin. Pract.* **2014**, *68*, 756–760. [CrossRef]
84. Argyriou, A.A.; Park, S.B.; Islam, B.; Tamburin, S.; Velasco, R.; Alberti, P.; Bruna, J.; Psimaras, D.; Cavaletti, G.; Cornblath, D.R. Neurophysiological, nerve imaging and other techniques to assess chemotherapy-induced peripheral neurotoxicity in the clinical and research settings. *J. Neurol. Neurosurg. Psychiatry* **2019**, jnnp-2019-320969. [CrossRef] [PubMed]
85. Saad, M.; Psimaras, D.; Tafani, C.; Sallansonnet-Froment, M.; Calvet, J.-H.; Vilier, A.; Tigaud, J.-M.; Bompaire, F.; Lebouteux, M.; de Greslan, F.; et al. Quick, non-invasive and quantitative assessment of small fiber neuropathy in patients receiving chemotherapy. *J. Neuroo.* **2016**, *127*, 373–380. [CrossRef]
86. Kamei, K.; Ohnishi, T.; Nakata, K.; Danno, K.; Ohkawa, A.; Miyake, Y.; Okazaki, S.; Fukunaga, M.; Toyokawa, A.; Hamada, T.; et al. A new monitoring tool CLIP test for progression of oxaliplatin-induced peripheral neuropathy: A multicenter prospective study. *Asia-Pac. J. Clin. Oncol.* **2020**, *16*. [CrossRef]
87. Park, S.B.; Lin, C.S.-Y.; Krishnan, A.V.; Goldstein, D.; Friedlander, M.L.; Kiernan, M.C. Utilizing natural activity to dissect the pathophysiology of acute oxaliplatin-induced neuropathy. *Exp. Neurol.* **2011**, *227*, 120–127. [CrossRef] [PubMed]

88. Kiernan, M.C.; Bostock, H.; Park, S.B.; Kaji, R.; Krarup, C.; Krishnan, A.V.; Kuwabara, S.; Lin, C.S.-Y.; Misawa, S.; Moldovan, M.; et al. Measurement of axonal excitability: Consensus guidelines. *Clin. Neuro.* **2020**, *131*, 308–323. [CrossRef] [PubMed]
89. Bennedsgaard, K.; Ventzel, L.; Grafe, P.; Tigerholm, J.; Themistocleous, A.C.; Bennett, D.L.; Tankisi, H.; Finnerup, N.B. Cold aggravates abnormal excitability of motor axons in oxaliplatin-treated patients. *Muscle Nerve* **2020**, *61*, 796–800. [CrossRef] [PubMed]
90. Park, S.B.; Lin, C.S.-Y.; Kiernan, M.C. Nerve Excitability Assessment in Chemotherapy-induced Neurotoxicity. *JoVE* **2012**, 3439. [CrossRef] [PubMed]
91. Park, S.B.; Goldstein, D.; Lin, C.S.-Y.; Krishnan, A.V.; Friedlander, M.L.; Kiernan, M.C. Acute Abnormalities of Sensory Nerve Function Associated With Oxaliplatin-Induced Neurotoxicity. *JCO* **2009**, *27*, 1243–1249. [CrossRef] [PubMed]
92. Koskinen, M.J.; Kautio, A.-L.; Haanpää, M.L.; Haapasalo, H.K.; Kellokumpu-Lehtinen, P.-L.; Saarto, T.; Hietaharju, A.J. Intraepidermal nerve fibre density in cancer patients receiving adjuvant chemotherapy. *Anticancer Res.* **2011**, *31*, 4413–4416. [PubMed]
93. Velasco, R.; Navarro, X.; Gil-Gil, M.; Herrando-Grabulosa, M.; Calls, A.; Bruna, J. Neuropathic Pain and Nerve Growth Factor in Chemotherapy-Induced Peripheral Neuropathy: Prospective Clinical-Pathological Study. *J. Pain Symptom. Manag.* **2017**, *54*, 815–825. [CrossRef] [PubMed]
94. Bonomo, R.; Cavaletti, G. Clinical and biochemical markers in CIPN: A reappraisal. *Rev. Neurol.* **2021**, S003537872100028X. [CrossRef]
95. Staff, N.P.; Cavaletti, G.; Islam, B.; Lustberg, M.; Psimaras, D.; Tamburin, S. Platinum-induced peripheral neurotoxicity: From pathogenesis to treatment. *J. Peripher. Nerv. Syst.* **2019**, *24*. [CrossRef]
96. Argyriou, A.A.; Bruna, J.; Genazzani, A.A.; Cavaletti, G. Chemotherapy-induced peripheral neurotoxicity: Management informed by pharmacogenetics. *Nat. Rev. Neurol.* **2017**, *13*, 492–504. [CrossRef]
97. Lecomte, T.; Landi, B.; Beaune, P.; Laurent-Puig, P.; Loriot, M.-A. Glutathione S-Transferase P1 Polymorphism (Ile [105] Val) Predicts Cumulative Neuropathy in Patients Receiving Oxaliplatin-Based Chemotherapy. *Clin. Cancer Res.* **2006**, *12*, 3050–3056. [CrossRef]
98. Kumamoto, K.; Ishibashi, K.; Okada, N.; Tajima, Y.; Kuwabara, K.; Kumagai, Y.; Baba, H.; Haga, N.; Ishida, H. Polymorphisms of GSTP1, ERCC2 and TS-3'UTR are associated with the clinical outcome of mFOLFOX6 in colorectal cancer patients. *Oncol. Lett.* **2013**, *6*, 648–654. [CrossRef]
99. Chen, Y.-C.; Tzeng, C.-H.; Chen, P.-M.; Lin, J.-K.; Lin, T.-C.; Chen, W.-S.; Jiang, J.-K.; Wang, H.-S.; Wang, W.-S. Influence of GSTP1 I105V polymorphism on cumulative neuropathy and outcome of FOLFOX-4 treatment in Asian patients with colorectal carcinoma. *Cancer Sci.* **2010**, *101*, 530–535. [CrossRef]
100. Liu, Y.-P.; Ling, Y.; Qi, Q.-F.; Zhang, Y.-P.; Zhang, C.-S.; Zhu, C.-T.; Wang, M.-H.; Pan, Y.-D. Genetic polymorphisms of ERCC1-118, XRCC1-399 and GSTP1-105 are associated with the clinical outcome of gastric cancer patients receiving oxaliplatin-based adjuvant chemotherapy. *Mol. Med. Rep.* **2013**, *7*, 1904–1911. [CrossRef]
101. Ruzzo, A.; Graziano, F.; Loupakis, F.; Rulli, E.; Canestrari, E.; Santini, D.; Catalano, V.; Ficarelli, R.; Maltese, P.; Bisonni, R.; et al. Pharmacogenetic Profiling in Patients With Advanced Colorectal Cancer Treated With First-Line FOLFOX-4 Chemotherapy. *JCO* **2007**, *25*, 1247–1254. [CrossRef]
102. McLeod, H.L.; Sargent, D.J.; Marsh, S.; Green, E.M.; King, C.R.; Fuchs, C.S.; Ramanathan, R.K.; Williamson, S.K.; Findlay, B.P.; Thibodeau, S.N.; et al. Pharmacogenetic Predictors of Adverse Events and Response to Chemotherapy in Metastatic Colorectal Cancer: Results From North American Gastrointestinal Intergroup Trial N9741. *JCO* **2010**, *28*, 3227–3233. [CrossRef] [PubMed]
103. Zarate, R.; Rodríguez, J.; Bandres, E.; Patiño-Garcia, A.; Ponz-Sarvise, M.; Viudez, A.; Ramirez, N.; Bitarte, N.; Chopitea, A.; Gacía-Foncillas, J. Oxaliplatin, irinotecan and capecitabine as first-line therapy in metastatic colorectal cancer (mCRC): A dose-finding study and pharmacogenomic analysis. *Br. J. Cancer* **2010**, *102*, 987–994. [CrossRef] [PubMed]
104. Boige, V.; Mendiboure, J.; Pignon, J.-P.; Loriot, M.-A.; Castaing, M.; Barrois, M.; Malka, D.; Trégouët, D.-A.; Bouché, O.; Le Corre, D.; et al. Pharmacogenetic Assessment of Toxicity and Outcome in Patients With Metastatic Colorectal Cancer Treated With LV5FU2, FOLFOX, and FOLFIRI: FFCD 2000-05. *JCO* **2010**, *28*, 2556–2564. [CrossRef] [PubMed]
105. Ruzzo, A.; Graziano, F.; Galli, F.; Giacomini, E.; Floriani, I.; Galli, F.; Rulli, E.; Lonardi, S.; Ronzoni, M.; Massidda, B.; et al. Genetic markers for toxicity of adjuvant oxaliplatin and fluoropyrimidines in the phase III TOSCA trial in high-risk colon cancer patients. *Sci. Rep.* **2014**, *4*, 6828. [CrossRef]
106. Custodio, A.; Moreno-Rubio, J.; Aparicio, J.; Gallego-Plazas, J.; Yaya, R.; Maurel, J.; Higuera, O.; Burgos, E.; Ramos, D.; Calatrava, A.; et al. Pharmacogenetic predictors of severe peripheral neuropathy in colon cancer patients treated with oxaliplatin-based adjuvant chemotherapy: A GEMCAD group study. *Ann. Oncol.* **2014**, *25*, 398–403. [CrossRef]
107. Kanai, M.; Kawaguchi, T.; Kotaka, M.; Shinozaki, K.; Touyama, T.; Manaka, D.; Ishigure, K.; Hasegawa, J.; Munemoto, Y.; Matsui, T.; et al. Large-scale prospective pharmacogenomics study of oxaliplatin-induced neuropathy in colon cancer patients enrolled in the JFMC41-1001-C2 (JOIN Trial). *Ann. Oncol.* **2016**, *27*, 1143–1148. [CrossRef]
108. Nichetti, F.; Falvella, F.S.; Miceli, R.; Cheli, S.; Gaetano, R.; Fucà, G.; Infante, G.; Martinetti, A.; Antoniotti, C.; Falcone, A.; et al. Is a pharmacogenomic panel useful to estimate the risk of oxaliplatin-related neurotoxicity in colorectal cancer patients? *Pharm. J.* **2019**, *19*, 465–472. [CrossRef]

109. Palugulla, S.; Devaraju, P.; Kayal, S.; Narayan, S.K.; Mathaiyan, J. Genetic polymorphisms in cyclin H gene are associated with oxaliplatin-induced acute peripheral neuropathy in South Indian digestive tract cancer patients. *Cancer Chemother. Pharm.* **2018**, *82*, 421–428. [CrossRef]
110. Lee, K.-H.; Chang, H.J.; Han, S.-W.; Oh, D.-Y.; Im, S.-A.; Bang, Y.-J.; Kim, S.Y.; Lee, K.-W.; Kim, J.H.; Hong, Y.S.; et al. Pharmacogenetic analysis of adjuvant FOLFOX for Korean patients with colon cancer. *Cancer Chemother. Pharm.* **2013**, *71*, 843–851. [CrossRef]
111. Cortejoso, L.; García, M.I.; García-Alfonso, P.; González-Haba, E.; Escolar, F.; Sanjurjo, M.; López-Fernández, L.A. Differential toxicity biomarkers for irinotecan- and oxaliplatin-containing chemotherapy in colorectal cancer. *Cancer Chemother. Pharm.* **2013**, *71*, 1463–1472. [CrossRef]
112. Cecchin, E.; D'Andrea, M.; Lonardi, S.; Zanusso, C.; Pella, N.; Errante, D.; De Mattia, E.; Polesel, J.; Innocenti, F.; Toffoli, G. A prospective validation pharmacogenomic study in the adjuvant setting of colorectal cancer patients treated with the 5-fluorouracil/leucovorin/oxaliplatin (FOLFOX4) regimen. *Pharm. J.* **2013**, *13*, 403–409. [CrossRef]
113. Argyriou, A.A.; Antonacopoulou, A.G.; Scopa, C.D.; Kottorou, A.; Kominea, A.; Peroukides, S.; Kalofonos, H.P. Liability of the Voltage-Gated Sodium Channel Gene *SCN2A* R19K Polymorphism to Oxaliplatin-Induced Peripheral Neuropathy. *Oncology* **2009**, *77*, 254–256. [CrossRef]
114. Argyriou, A.A.; Cavaletti, G.; Antonacopoulou, A.; Genazzani, A.A.; Briani, C.; Bruna, J.; Terrazzino, S.; Velasco, R.; Alberti, P.; Campagnolo, M.; et al. Voltage-gated sodium channel polymorphisms play a pivotal role in the development of oxaliplatin-induced peripheral neurotoxicity: Results from a prospective multicenter study. *Cancer* **2013**, *119*, 3570–3577. [CrossRef] [PubMed]
115. Sereno, M.; Gutiérrez-Gutiérrez, G.; Rubio, J.M.; Apellániz-Ruiz, M.; Sánchez-Barroso, L.; Casado, E.; Falagan, S.; López-Gómez, M.; Merino, M.; Gómez-Raposo, C.; et al. Genetic polymorphisms of SCN9A are associated with oxaliplatin-induced neuropathy. *BMC Cancer* **2017**, *17*, 63. [CrossRef] [PubMed]
116. Basso, M.; Modoni, A.; Spada, D.; Cassano, A.; Schinzari, G.; Lo Monaco, M.; Quaranta, D.; Tonali, P.A.; Barone, C. Polymorphism of CAG motif of SK3 gene is associated with acute oxaliplatin neurotoxicity. *Cancer Chemother. Pharm.* **2011**, *67*, 1179–1187. [CrossRef]
117. Anon, B.; Largeau, B.; Girault, A.; Chantome, A.; Caulet, M.; Perray, C.; Moussata, D.; Vandier, C.; Barin-Le Guellec, C.; Lecomte, T. Possible association of CAG repeat polymorphism in KCNN3 encoding the potassium channel SK3 with oxaliplatin-induced neurotoxicity. *Cancer Chemother. Pharm.* **2018**, *82*, 149–157. [CrossRef] [PubMed]
118. Argyriou, A.A.; Park, S.B.; Bruna, J.; Cavaletti, G. Voltage-gated sodium channel dysfunction and the search for other satellite channels in relation to acute oxaliplatin-induced peripheral neurotoxicity. *J. Peripher. Nerv. Syst.* **2019**, *24*, 360–361. [CrossRef] [PubMed]
119. Won, H.-H.; Lee, J.; Park, J.O.; Park, Y.S.; Lim, H.Y.; Kang, W.K.; Kim, J.-W.; Lee, S.-Y.; Park, S.H. Polymorphic markers associated with severe oxaliplatin-induced, chronic peripheral neuropathy in colon cancer patients. *Cancer* **2012**, *118*, 2828–2836. [CrossRef]
120. Terrazzino, S.; Argyriou, A.A.; Cargnin, S.; Antonacopoulou, A.G.; Briani, C.; Bruna, J.; Velasco, R.; Alberti, P.; Campagnolo, M.; Lonardi, S.; et al. Genetic determinants of chronic oxaliplatin-induced peripheral neurotoxicity: A genome-wide study replication and meta-analysis. *J. Peripher. Nerv. Syst.* **2015**, *20*, 15–23. [CrossRef]
121. Adjei, A.A.; Lopez, C.L.; Schaid, D.J.; Sloan, J.A.; Le-Rademacher, J.G.; Loprinzi, C.L.; Norman, A.D.; Olson, J.E.; Couch, F.J.; Beutler, A.S.; et al. Genetic Predictors of Chemotherapy-Induced Peripheral Neuropathy from Paclitaxel, Carboplatin and Oxaliplatin: NCCTG/Alliance N08C1, N08CA and N08CB Study. *Cancers* **2021**, *13*, 1084. [CrossRef]
122. Loucks, C.M.; Yan, K.; Tanoshima, R.; Ross, C.J.D.; Rassekh, S.R.; Carleton, B.C. Pharmacogenetic testing to guide therapeutic decision-making and improve outcomes for children undergoing anthracycline-based chemotherapy. *Basic Clin. Pharm. Toxicol* **2021**, bcpt.13593. [CrossRef]
123. Meulendijks, D.; Henricks, L.M.; Sonke, G.S.; Deenen, M.J.; Froehlich, T.K.; Amstutz, U.; Largiadèr, C.R.; Jennings, B.A.; Marinaki, A.M.; Sanderson, J.D.; et al. Clinical relevance of DPYD variants c.1679T>G, c.1236G>A/HapB3, and c.1601G>A as predictors of severe fluoropyrimidine-associated toxicity: A systematic review and meta-analysis of individual patient data. *Lancet Oncol.* **2015**, *16*, 1639–1650. [CrossRef]
124. Briani, C.; Campagnolo, M.; Lucchetta, M.; Cacciavillani, M.; Dalla Torre, C.; Granata, G.; Bergamo, F.; Lonardi, S.; Zagonel, V.; Cavaletti, G.; et al. Ultrasound assessment of oxaliplatin-induced neuropathy and correlations with neurophysiologic findings. *Eur. J. Neurol.* **2013**, *20*, 188–192. [CrossRef] [PubMed]
125. Pitarokoili, K.; Höffken, N.; Lönneker, N.; Fisse, A.L.; Trampe, N.; Gold, R.; Reinacher-Schick, A.; Yoon, M.-S. Prospective Study of the Clinical, Electrophysiologic, and Sonographic Characteristics of Oxaliplatin-Induced Neuropathy: HRUS in Oxaliplatin-Induced Neuropathy. *J. Neuroimaging* **2019**, *29*, 133–139. [CrossRef]
126. Campagnolo, M.; Lazzarini, D.; Fregona, I.; Cacciavillani, M.; Bergamo, F.; Parrozzani, R.; Midena, E.; Briani, C. Corneal confocal microscopy in patients with oxaliplatin-induced peripheral neuropathy. *J. Peripher. Nerv. Syst.* **2013**, *18*, 269–271. [CrossRef]
127. Ferdousi, M.; Azmi, S.; Petropoulos, I.N.; Fadavi, H.; Ponirakis, G.; Marshall, A.; Tavakoli, M.; Malik, I.; Mansoor, W.; Malik, R.A. Corneal Confocal Microscopy Detects Small Fibre Neuropathy in Patients with Upper Gastrointestinal Cancer and Nerve Regeneration in Chemotherapy Induced Peripheral Neuropathy. *PLoS ONE* **2015**, *10*, e0139394. [CrossRef] [PubMed]

128. Ali, R.; Baracos, V.E.; Sawyer, M.B.; Bianchi, L.; Roberts, S.; Assenat, E.; Mollevi, C.; Senesse, P. Lean body mass as an independent determinant of dose-limiting toxicity and neuropathy in patients with colon cancer treated with FOLFOX regimens. *Cancer Med.* **2016**, *5*, 607–616. [CrossRef]
129. El Chediak, A.; Haydar, A.; Hakim, A.; Abdel Massih, S.; Hilal, L.; Mukherji, D.; Temraz, S.; Shamseddine, A. Increase in spleen volume as a predictor of oxaliplatin toxicity. *TCRM* **2018**, *14*, 653–657. [CrossRef] [PubMed]
130. Pelosi, L.; Han, C.H.; McKeage, M.J. Muscle ultrasound in the assessment of oxaliplatin-induced neurotoxicity. *Clin. Neurophysiol.* **2020**, *131*, 343–344. [CrossRef]
131. Khalil, M.; Teunissen, C.E.; Otto, M.; Piehl, F.; Sormani, M.P.; Gattringer, T.; Barro, C.; Kappos, L.; Comabella, M.; Fazekas, F.; et al. Neurofilaments as biomarkers in neurological disorders. *Nat. Rev. Neurol.* **2018**, *14*, 577–589. [CrossRef]
132. Meregalli, C.; Fumagalli, G.; Alberti, P.; Canta, A.; Carozzi, V.A.; Chiorazzi, A.; Monza, L.; Pozzi, E.; Sandelius, Å.; Blennow, K.; et al. Neurofilament light chain as disease biomarker in a rodent model of chemotherapy induced peripheral neuropathy. *Exp. Neurol.* **2018**, *307*, 129–132. [CrossRef] [PubMed]
133. Kim, S.-H.; Choi, M.K.; Park, N.Y.; Hyun, J.-W.; Lee, M.Y.; Kim, H.J.; Jung, S.K.; Cha, Y. Serum neurofilament light chain levels as a biomarker of neuroaxonal injury and severity of oxaliplatin-induced peripheral neuropathy. *Sci. Rep.* **2020**, *10*, 7995. [CrossRef] [PubMed]
134. Cavaletti, G.; Petruccioli, M.G.; Marmiroli, P.; Rigolio, R.; Galbiati, S.; Zoia, C.; Ferrarese, C.; Tagliabue, E.; Dolci, C.; Bayssas, M.; et al. Circulating nerve growth factor level changes during oxaliplatin treatment-induced neurotoxicity in the rat. *Anticancer Res.* **2002**, *22*, 4199–4204. [PubMed]

MDPI
St. Alban-Anlage 66
4052 Basel
Switzerland
Tel. +41 61 683 77 34
Fax +41 61 302 89 18
www.mdpi.com

Journal of Personalized Medicine Editorial Office
E-mail: jpm@mdpi.com
www.mdpi.com/journal/jpm

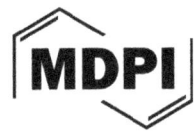

www.ingramcontent.com/pod-product-compliance
Lightning Source LLC
LaVergne TN
LVHW070558100526
838202LV00012B/503